Human Forever

Searching the World for a Better Life with Dementia

Teun Toebes &
Jonathan de Jong

Translated by Laura Vroomen

s
ept
em
b
er

First published in the United Kingdom by September in 2026

September, an imprint of Duckworth Books Ltd
1 Golden Court, Richmond, TW9 1EU, United Kingdom
www.septemberpublishing.org

First published in the Dutch language by De Arbeiderspers, Amsterdam
Original title: *Een Wereld te Winnen*

A catalogue record for this book is available from the British Library

Photos: Jonathan de Jong, stills from the documentary *Human Forever*
Typography: Perfect Service

Printed and bound in Great Britain by Clays Ltd, Elcograf S.p.A.

The authorised representative in the EEA is Easy Access System Europe, Mustamäe tee 50, 10621 Tallinn, Estonia.

1

Paperback ISBN: 9780715656570
eISBN: 9780715656587

MIX
Paper | Supporting responsible forestry
FSC® C018072

Teun Toebes, dubbed the 'Greta Thunberg of healthcare', started his career in nursing and care ethics. He evolved into an international healthcare innovator who fights to improve the quality of life for people touched by dementia across the globe. He has received many awards and is a popular speaker at international conferences and in the media. His previous book, *The Housemates*, was translated into English, German, Italian and Arabic and was a number one bestseller in the Netherlands. teuntoebes.com

Jonathan de Jong is a multi-award-winning documentary filmmaker and bestselling author. His work is characterised by social and human stories that are highly impactful. Together with Teun Toebes, he wrote *The Housemates* and created the international hit documentary *Human Forever.*

Praise for *The Housemates*:

'[*The Housemates*] not only celebrates the joy of this particular form of intergenerational living, but irradiates the often-grim truth of life in Western dementia care… a lovely and humane book' ***Telegraph***

'A young Dutchman's compelling account of his decision to move into a care home shines a light on a system that erodes self-worth' ***Observer***

'There are plenty of uplifting and charming moments at Friday night drinks and chats with his new eighty and ninety-something friends, as they swap notes on clothes, their love lives and their lives before. But there is real urgency at the core of this book' ***The Times***

'Captivating' ***Daily Express***

'Celebrates the joy of intergenerational living, and questions whether we might treat old people differently' ***Fabulous Magazine***

Also by Teun Toebes and Jonathan de Jong:

The Housemates: Everything One Young Student Learnt about Love, Care and Dementia from Living in a Nursing Home

'The key thing to remember is that up until the very end people with dementia have feelings and a rich inner life.'
- Carla Molenberghs

Contents

Foreword

My name is Teun. I'm 24, in perfect health and I live in the secure unit of a nursing home.

Why?

I'm 24, but I won't be forever...

Right now, people still listen to what I want,
what I feel and what I think.
Right now, I still have the freedom to be who I am and go where I please,
but there's a one-in-five chance that this won't be the case in the future.

So I'm going in search of answers for later.

Now that I've been living in a nursing home for several years, I'm seeing how 'normal' life is gradually seeping away under the locked door. That really gets to my housemates, leaving them with a sense of isolation and exclusion, with a feeling that they 'no longer matter'. With each passing day, their sad-ness weighs heavier on me. I can't imagine that this was the life we envisioned for people living with dementia when we created this form of institutional care. How did we get here and, more importantly, how can we change it?

To answer that big question, I decided, three years ago, to travel the world with my good friend, filmmaker Jonathan de Jong, to investigate the situation elsewhere. How do other countries deal with dementia? What kind of care do they offer to people living with the condition? Why this particular approach? What new developments or insights do they have? And most importantly: what can we learn from one another in our bid to provide a more humane future for all people with some form of dementia and their nearest and dearest? Given that the number of dementia sufferers is set to double in the next 20 years (to an estimated 81 million worldwide by 2040), such an exploration is vital.

Not long after we started our research, we came across an international agreement on a good standard of living. Drawn up a long time ago, Article 25 of the Universal Declaration of Human Rights describes a life that me and my housemates are not fully experiencing at the moment.

> Everyone has the right to a standard of living adequate for the health and well-being of himself and of his family, including food, clothing, housing and medical care and necessary social services, and the right to security in the event of unemployment, sickness, disability, widowhood, old age or other lack of livelihood in circumstances beyond his control.

With this article in the back of our minds, we went in search of what really defines compassion and coexistence. We were curious to see if, on an international level, we are all sticking to our agreements. Are we still looking after one another? And how do the people who need care experience this? Because if there's one thing I've learnt it's this: dementia is usually talked about in terms of loss, but there's still a world to be won.

Expected global increase in dementia

Expected increase in dementia, worldwide 2019-2050

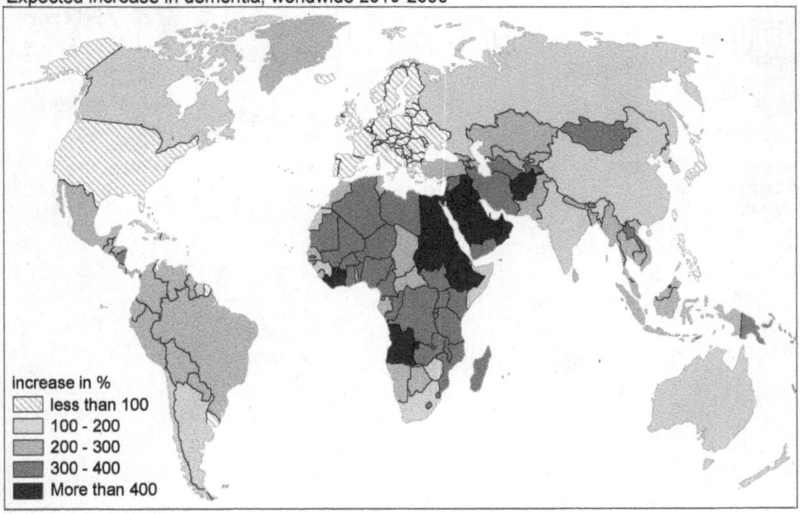

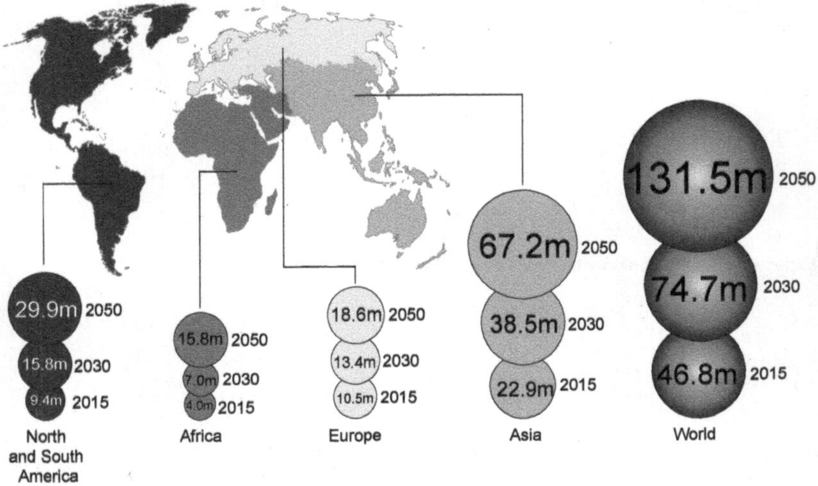
29.9m 2050
15.8m 2030
9.4m 2015
North and South America
15.8m 2050
7.0m 2030
4.0m 2015
Africa
18.6m 2050
13.4m 2030
10.5m 2015
Europe
67.2m 2050
38.5m 2030
22.9m 2015
Asia
131.5m 2050
74.7m 2030
46.8m 2015
World

I Status quo

The start of a quest

Utrecht, the Netherlands

'Mate...? Mate?' I'm just getting dressed when I hear frantic calls from the corridor.

I quickly pull on a jumper. 'Yes, Ad, what is it? I'm in my room.'

There's the instantly recognisable sound of my friend's orthopaedic shoes shuffling down the corridor, like a broom across gravel. This has been happening about ten times a day lately, as Ad seems to sense that I'm nearing the end of my stay here.

'Gosh, lad, am I pleased to see you! You've been away so much. You're not leaving us, are you?' He leans against the door frame, huffing and puffing, to recover from his early morning exertions.

'No, Ad, not yet... But as you know, I won't be here forever, and I'm finding it harder and harder to keep going. How about a cuppa?'

I don't want to lie to Ad, but it's not easy. I'm constantly trying to strike a balance between being honest with him and not needlessly hurting him, because I know that changes make him anxious. It would be hard for him to lose the support he has in me. His dementia further complicates the situation, because his sense of time is worsening and he's getting things mixed up. Not that long ago, he walked into my room all suited and booted to attend the premiere of my theatre show, which had taken place the previous month. I'll never forget the intense sadness on his face when the penny dropped. 'Oops, here we go again,' he said, before turning round with his shoulders slumped and dragging his freshly shined shoes back across the equally shiny linoleum floor to his room. These are the moments that make my life here really tough, and the mere thought of upsetting Ad fills me with guilt.

'But, eh, yeah, glad you're not leaving, buddy. Are you coming round to my room for a pint tonight?' Ad asks, clearly reassured, and knocks back his coffee in one go, which is what he likes to do with his beer as well.

'Of course, Ad, sounds great.' As he walks out the door, I add: 'Is there football on telly?'

From the corridor he yells back in his inimitable style: 'There's always football on telly, lad...'

With a grin on my face I put on my coat, grab my laptop and run to get my bike to make it to my lecture on time. When I cross the Oudegracht with sweat pouring down my back, I think to myself: my mind is made up, I'm moving out!

Ever since my book *The Housemates* was published in 2021, the atmosphere in the nursing home has been strained, a bit like an unspoken family feud. The carers are friendly enough to my face, but their body language speaks volumes: back off! I understand where they're coming from and it's certainly no surprise, but it is getting to me. I've never felt lonelier or more apprehensive about walking onto a ward, because I feel that the suffocating silence could erupt into a storm at any time. And none of it is made any easier by TV crews and newspaper journalists turning up every other day to catch 'that cute lad' living at the nursing home.

So it comes as a huge relief when a carer with whom I've built up a relationship of trust asks if I'm happy with the book's impact.

'Finally! I'm so glad you ask, Niels,' I say, and my voice breaks.

'Hey, no need to get all emotional,' he tries to put me at ease. 'I think it's a brave thing to do, you know, putting your finger on the sore spot while you're living here. Of course, people are a bit upset, but it'll pass... I know it's nothing personal but try explaining that to someone who's been working here for the past thirty years trying to do the best job possible and now suddenly they have this mirror held up to them.' He's clearly doing his best to get the message across in the nicest possible way. 'It's very simple: this is your home and day in day out you see everybody here waiting for the end. You owe it to yourself to speak up. I'd love it if I didn't have to follow a care plan, check things off a list or monitor stools, so I'd have more time to spend with people. I'm behind you, all the way. So keep it up. I'll talk them round... Here, have a cup of that weak filter coffee you mentioned in your book.'

As the weeks pass and the first wave of attention dies down, one thought stays with me: I need to show more clearly that change is possible. The many questions and reactions I receive suggest to me that people are happy to accept that a different outlook leads to a different outcome, but they struggle to imagine what that might be. What we really need are more answers. One day, it suddenly dawns on me that I need to roll up my sleeves and head out into the world.

Energised by this light-bulb moment, I take a bowl of olives out of the fridge and leg it to Muriëlle to tell her about my brilliant idea, because if there's anyone who appreciates an adventure it's her. Along with Ad, Leny, Tineke and Elly, she's one of my best friends in the nursing home. Muriëlle and I can natter endlessly about the big topics, like global warming and politics, as well as the little, more domestic ones and our other housemates. Gossip, you might call it. Like some kind of judge on wheels, she's quick to give her verdict on noisy neighbours, bossy sisters and pushy men. It makes any visit with her an absolute joy.

'Muriëlle, I have news!' I yell as I charge into her room. 'Muri...' That's when I see the pale, sunken face. She's normally so radiant, this woman from the Dutch Antilles. 'Are you not feeling well?' I ask, much more muted this time, and sit down on the edge of her bed.

'No, Teun... I miss life and company. My daughter Rosita visits a lot, but I still feel isolated. When you're not around, I just sit and stare into space, daydreaming about what used to be. I don't think that's what the end of life is supposed to be like, do you?'

I get the impression that she's saying goodbye, but I don't know what shape it's going to take.

'And that's why, dear Teun – this is really difficult for me to say, because I'm going to miss you terribly – I'm thinking of moving. To somewhere near Harderwijk, to be closer to my daughter.'

Although I'm relieved we're not talking about the other type of farewell, which I was worried about for a moment, I'm not sure what to make of this surprise. I just sit in silence.

Muriëlle takes my hand. 'You ought to consider it yourself... But anyway, what was it you were so eager to tell me a minute ago?'

However much I'd love to admit that, like her, I'm thinking of moving, I don't want to steal her thunder. At the same time, I wonder if what she's telling me is true and whether it's feasible, but I choose to do what I always do: go along and believe the other person until proven wrong.

I get pissed off with myself when I notice that I question what my housemates are saying, because at that particular moment in time it doesn't really matter whether it's true or not, and I always want to do right by them. There's the pitfall that your 'factual' truth eclipses the 'emotional' truth of what someone with dementia is trying to tell you. And if there's one thing I've learnt from my housemates is that emotion is the lifeblood of the secure unit. By reading the emotion underlying the behaviour, you find out what's true and valuable to the person you're interacting with.

Before Muriëlle pops not an olive but a garlic clove into her mouth, she presses me: 'Well? How about it, young man? What was so urgent?'

'I came to tell you that I want to travel the world to explore how other countries deal with dementia, how people elsewhere live their lives and what we can learn from them. How cool is that?'

She looks dubious. 'You? Travel the world all by yourself?'

'No, probably with the documentary maker who came over for coffee not that long ago...' I'm bluffing, because I haven't actually discussed the plan with Jonathan yet, but I know it's not a bad idea. We click, because we share a love for people with dementia and we're keen to improve their world.

Her beady black eyes are gleaming. 'Oh, you mean the tall guy with the cap?' She may be losing track of time and events, but her dementia has done nothing to erode her interest in men.

'Yes, that's the one!' I say.

Looking pleased with herself, she pricks two olives onto her pick. 'It's nice that the two of you want to do that. Useful, too. A bit of youthful energy wouldn't go amiss round here...'

Ever since I moved in, Muriëlle has been my compass. She always knows just what to say and sometimes she even intuits things that are still unspoken in my mind. Truly remarkable. These are the everyday moments that I cherish and that I want to show to the outside world, because it's not something that people see. It's precisely by sharing such experiences that you do right by a group that has so much to say yet is so rarely heard.

To turn my wild idea into reality, I decide to call Jonathan straight after my chat with Muriëlle. He doesn't beat about the bush: 'Yes, amazing! Let's discuss it soon and start planning. This could turn into something very special...'

Jonathan's interest in the subject dates back to his student days, when for six years he had a part-time job driving people with dementia to and from a daycare centre. In between drives, he'd clean on the secure unit. The world he saw left a lasting impression on him, and as a freelance filmmaker he decided to make it the subject of a documentary series. It was well-received in the Netherlands and even won an award, prompting the manager of the care farm that featured in the documentary to bring us together for a film. It turned out to be a match made in heaven. Thank you again, Francien!

A week later we're sitting at the table in my room to seal the deal. We decide to explore how the lives of people with dementia can be improved. It's important that we do this with an open mind and not let ourselves be blinded by the self-image that 'the Dutch provide the best care in the world'. That's not the impression I've been getting from my housemates and their families these past few years. It's a bitter truth that people with dementia are never really taken into consideration when such claims are made, even though they're always wheeled out for smiley pictures on nursing home websites like some sort of advertisement for our superior care.

Thanks to these images, hinting at a long and happy life, many families view a nursing home as an oasis of peace and quiet, somewhere safe where they can leave their loved one without a guilty conscience. But they usually don't stop to ask what exactly makes a happy life and whether their loved one actually *wants* to be safe behind lock and key. A poster or website featuring people with bruises would probably be a rather gruesome sight, but it would definitely be more realistic. At least it wouldn't depict the nursing home and the care it provides as some kind of health spa, and it would raise the key question of where a real life begins or ends, and who carries responsibility for it.

I really think we ought to paint a more truthful picture of care – of care in general, but especially during the later stages of life. I've noticed that it's a no-go area for just about everyone except my housemates. There's no such thing as privacy on a secure unit; you can't be self-conscious if you want your arse wiped, and death is a more frequent visitor than you'd like. It may not be the most appealing ad but imagine the disappointment when you find out that your fancy five-star resort is in fact a sad holiday camp without water slides that you can never leave.

Dropping a loved one off at a new home is tough enough, so let's agree not to make it worse by creating unrealistic expectations. Care providers don't want to disappoint families, and equally, families don't want to be disappointed, but in reality that's a common occurrence. We must ask ourselves in all seriousness whether it's possible to meet the wishes and expectations of those who have to live here. Perhaps that will finally bring us to a point where we can legitimately use those smiling photos.

We're both proactive people, so later that same week Jonathan is already filming in our living room. Our quest has officially begun.

Ad is fascinated by it all and keeps calling Jonathan 'director'. He must be impressed by all the camera equipment. 'Hey director,' he shouts from his regular place at the dining room table, 'are you guys filming in my room later? I can show you my Ministeck collection.'

Shortly after, we find ourselves in his room, which is full of boxes and plastic pegboards with depictions of tigers, landscapes and cartoon characters.

'Wow, impressive,' Jonathan says straight off.

A big grin spreads across Ad's face. 'Yes, it's taken me quite a bit of time...' He sits down at his desk and heaves a deep sigh.

'What's up, Ad?' I ask. 'Aren't you proud?'

He mutters something inaudible before he speaks up. 'Sure... maybe it's impressive, but it's just a way to pass the time, you know. The real world is outside, in here you're cooped up, so what are you going to do?'

Surprised by the sudden turn that this conversation has taken, Jonathan and I look at each other. Maybe the Ministeck collection was just an excuse and Ad lured us to his room because he wanted to air his grievances. 'Is that what it feels like?' I ask to encourage him to elaborate.

'It's true, right?' he says in a huff. 'I think it's a shame. All you can do is daydream. You can't go out. That's to say...,' he frowns and makes quote marks with his fingers.

'You mean you have to ask for permission?'

The look on his face speaks volumes. He stares at the floor and nods his head. 'Yeah, that can be hard. There's nothing else to do. If I didn't have this, then...' He points to his Misteck. 'Good riddance is what it feels like to me. And then they've got the gall to say: "He's got a good life in there." Convenient, that's what it is.'

Still unsettled by the words of my best friend in this home, I watch as he nods off in front of the television in his bedroom. It's showing commercials for sun-drenched holidays on exotic islands, and the contrast with this place couldn't be greater. In fact, in here it feels as if the outside world, as a whole, is something you only see on the box, the greenery beyond the tall fence as far away as these tropical destinations. My head is spinning. Is it true what Ad is saying? Is convenience really why we collectively lock people away in homes where only a meal or a carer might break up the monotony a bit? Surely that's not right?

I jump when I hear a voice from the kitchen behind me: 'Mr van Dokkum, Mr van Dokkum!'

Ad is startled too. He looks up and reacts like only he can: 'Whoa, where's the fire? I'm not deaf, you know?' When he sees me, he winks.

'You're funny. I wasn't sure if you were sleeping, but would you like another coffee?' the carer asks sweetly.

'Goes without saying. White with sugar,' Ad replies. He sits up a bit straighter in his chair again and grabs the remote. 'Let's see who's playing tonight.'

Intrigued by what Ad has told us, we decide to film in my home for a few weeks while we work out the international side of our research. We draw on everything we've learnt and appeal to everybody we know in the field of dementia to get an idea of what our adventure might look like. Before long, we realise that a global quest sounds great, but that carrying it out is a rather more complicated affair. Where to start? What countries and continents to include, and why? And more importantly: how do we get there?

In the months that follow, we speak to leading scientists, care organisations and others working in the area, which gives us a better understanding of the care system in the Netherlands and what we might learn in other countries. Eventually, the Ministry of Health, Welfare and Sport gets wind of our plans, and after several conversations about the increasing numbers of people with dementia and how to deal with them the ministry says it wants to support our trip and plans to include the resulting film in a G20 summit on dementia. With their backing, our research gains momentum. The world now feels within reach, and in a short space of time we make contact with government officials, scientists and other individuals from more than thirty-five countries.

Let me be clear: even a worldwide study can never capture the full truth, and that isn't the aim of our trip either. We're hoping to find answers that will help improve the quality of life for people with dementia; which country has the best health care, at least on paper, is less important to us. I believe it's something you need to experience first-hand, because during my stay in one of the world's best healthcare systems I've learnt that quality of life can never be quantified or qualified on the basis of figures alone. So as not to fall into that trap, we don't practise investigative journalism based on hard facts, but instead look at experiences from a human perspective.

So when the phone rings and I hear that we get to have such experiences somewhere, I immediately call Jonathan. 'We're off! Our trip is about to begin.'

'Cool! Where are we going first?' is his equally enthusiastic response.

'Apeldoorn,' I say with all the bravado I can muster.

This is met with silence. 'Apeldoorn, as in, barely 50 miles from here?'

'That's the one!'

'Great, I've always wanted to go!'

11 The poverty behind the prosperity

The 18 billion euro system that very few want to live in

Apeldoorn, the Netherlands

Carers often tell me: 'Teun, our home does care so much better. You really ought to come and have a look here.' But when I turn up at those places, I find that in most cases the very same care has simply been packaged in a different way. New buildings, sensory walls, hypermodern lighting and trendy furniture are all very well, but who decides what constitutes better care when you still have residents who are nodding off at the table or who don't have the strength to drag themselves to the fake bus stop or the multi-sensory room? How can we be proud of material things when all they really do is fool people or render them more passive? Sometimes it looks as if we're trying to create a playground for people with dementia and come up with all manner of activities to entertain 'them', so they don't realise how dismal their home is. Let's face it, we wouldn't want to spend our lives in a glorified ball pit either. Luckily, more and more places in the Netherlands are now making an effort to create a real home, but they're still the exceptions that prove the rule.

This picture was reinforced once more when I approached a friend and care administrator, Margje Mahler, and asked her if we could stay at one of her facilities for our documentary. Her immediate response was, 'Sure, but I'll show you a "standard home", because it would be too easy to score a quick win with one of our new small-scale locations. You see that a lot in the media these days.' She gave me a look as if to say, 'right?'

That's cool, I thought. Putting yourself and your organisation in a vulnerable position because you want to contribute to the progress that's so desperately needed.

'Small-scale places are great,' she resumed, 'but the vast majority of people in our country wind up in large nursing homes. So if we really want to achieve change we must look at how we can turn those large-scale institutions into places where people actually feel at home.' Margje told me that she already had a location in mind for us, with the promising name Het Zonnehuis, or The Sun House. Situated in the village of Beekbergen, not far from Apeldoorn, it is the oldest nursing home in the country. 'It has been refurbished a few times since 1929, but now we're in the process of looking how we might future proof it. If the two of you get your things ready, I'll give everybody a heads up so you can move in soon.'

Just over a month later, I'm driving my old banger through the forest-rich landscape of the Veluwe region when something that looks unmistakably like a nursing home looms up at the end of the road. In the bright sunshine, the contrast between the original and the more modern buildings that have been added over the years is as sharp as can be. Jonathan is waiting for me as I pull up in the large, paved car park. I cut the engine and grab my duffel bag with clothes from behind the passenger seat.

We're excited as we walk through a sliding door towards reception, where we receive a warm welcome. Together with a member of staff we head to the ward and, along the way, stop in front of Jo Visser's portrait. Ironically, it hangs above the keypad that provides access to the world that she helped create. Jo is one of the founding mothers of the nursing home in general, and Het Zonnehuis in particular. And now, nearly a hundred years later, I'm visiting her brainchild to see if this is still the best way to organise care.

Shortly afterwards, we have to negotiate yet another locked door, and behind this one we find two residents who've barricaded themselves, intent on escaping. So it's the same story here, I think, and try to make contact with them to ease the suffering. When something like this happens at my nursing home, it always cuts me to the quick, not just because the people tend to have this fearful look in their eyes, but also because of what's being said to calm them down: 'It's alright, Mrs Hendriks, you're not in Hoenderloo, you're living here. Your father will be visiting shortly. No, you'll get to see your children later. Now be a "good girl" and come along to the living room.' You don't have to be a rocket scientist to understand that the residents don't usually fall for that, and it only adds fuel to the fire. In those cases, the screams can be heard echoing through the long corridors. Heart-rending.

It's actually very simple: no matter how old or new a location is, you're always aware that you're locked up. During a brief visit to the world-famous Hogeweyk dementia village, which was designed as a kind of gated community for people with the condition, I witnessed the exact same thing: people behind closed doors who wanted to leave. Whatever you call the gate to the outside world and wherever you place it, our innate desire for freedom will always manage to locate it.

Nursing home care in the Netherlands has an annual budget of more than 18 billion euros, which amounts to an average of around 1,000 euros per citizen per year. Is this what an 18 billion system has to offer us? Can we really not create more happiness with all that money?

After the 'escapees' have been escorted back to the house and we've introduced ourselves to the carers, I head to my room at the end of the dark corridor with its green linoleum flooring. The fancy castle gate print on my door, which the staff had been bragging about earlier, feels like a commentary on the secure fortress I find myself in, and the hospital bed – complete with lifting pole – doesn't do much to cheer me up either. For a change, I decide to neatly store the contents of my duffel bag in the designated wardrobe space.

Imagine that this isn't a slumber party, as it is for us, but you've just moved here permanently. Wouldn't you feel rather deflated? Especially when you realise that the room's only saving grace is the welcome card with sunflowers on your bedside cabinet. This isn't how you'd picture a warm and loving home, right? I bet none of the staff here would want this place for themselves or a loved one, so why do they think it's OK to work here? Sitting on the bed, staring at the tall steel fence around the inner courtyard, I decide to ask them.

When I've pulled myself together, I make my way to the living room, where I'm welcomed by the Drake of the nursing home world: Andre Rieu. Everywhere I go, I see the man playing endless waltzes on TVs that are never switched off. Unlike the residents at the back of the living room – they certainly are in sleep mode. With three of them slumped motionless with their heads on the table, the place looks more like a crime scene than a cosy break room. Again, this is more rule than exception in nursing homes. It's not André's fault, but when you're just sitting all day not even 'The Second Waltz' will keep you awake.

Thankfully, I hear a woman behind me ask me in a halting voice: 'T-tell me, who are you? And what are you doing here?'

I turn around and walk to the table where two ladies are sitting side by side. From the back, they could easily pass for sisters, with their short grey 'dos, floral blouses, black trousers and slip-ons. This is reinforced when I reach the table and see that the women, who are well into their eighties, don't just have identical glasses, but also the same curious look in their eyes. I plonk down on a chair and say: 'Let me introduce myself: my name is Teun, and I'm spending the weekend here.'

Her eyes widen and light up. 'Is that right? That makes you the second man here. The other one's Piet and he normally sits over there...'

Her jaunty demeanour immediately lifts my somewhat sombre mood. 'What's your name?' I ask.

She glances at her neighbour before telling me in a dignified manner: 'My name is Gon, and this here is Wil. But... how old are you?'

I look at the two eighty-plus ladies, who lean forward to hear my answer. 'Twenty-one.'

To be honest, I was counting on an 'Oh, really?', but after a brief silence, Gon simply says: 'Mmh, yes, I thought so. Nice, a few more men in the house.' I couldn't have wished for a better reaction. My peers often give me funny looks when I tell them that I live with older people, but Gon seems to think it's perfectly normal.

'I'm getting a bit peckish. Do you happen to know what time we're eating, ladies?' I ask, with an eye on the antique clock on the wall.

'At five o'clock sharp, lad. And you can stay where you are now. It's where Marie used to sit, but she's no longer with us... Lia is sitting next to you, and we're opposite you, okay?'

I nod to accept her seating arrangement. 'Yes, ma'am.'

She turns to face Wil, who moves a bit closer and cups her hand behind her ear to hear better. 'Right, we've got that all sewn up, Wil. Piet will be jealous...'

And while the ladies have a chuckle about their new table conquest, I slump a little and close my eyes for a quick nap, because 'When in Rome, do as the Romans do. Take it away, André...'

Slowly, the hubbub around me grows louder, and when I open my eyes and see that the table has been set I realise that I must have actually fallen asleep.

'Did you have a nice nap?' I'm asked by a member of staff who's putting the last few cups on the table.

'Eh, yes... I think so,' I say, still in a bit of a daze.

'I hope you like good old meat and two veg, because we're having beef roll with baked beans and salad.'

I'm not sure about this combination, but that doesn't stop me from replying with a wholehearted: 'Sounds great! When I'm at home I usually keep it simple too, so I'll be fine.'

That same moment a petite Dutch-Indonesian woman turns up in a bathrobe that's so thick it nearly doubles her in size. 'Hello young man. I spotted you earlier, but didn't want to wake you. I'm Lia, your neighbour at the table.' Right away, I notice her kind eyes as well as her way with words.

'Hello Lia, I'm Teun. How lovely to meet you. Come, let me get your chair for you.'

She bursts out laughing and rebuffs my bid to help. 'Don't be silly. I may be living in a nursing home, but I'm perfectly capable of doing that myself.' With her somewhat sarcastic tone, she reminds me of Muriëlle, whose sense of humour really livens things up in my unit, but which isn't appreciated by everyone.

Our neighbours across the table, who've just joined us, have their answer ready for Lia. Again, it evokes home. 'You might want to be a bit kinder to our newcomer, you know,' says Gon, who takes me under her maternal wing. 'Pay her no mind, boy. She doesn't really like it here. Oh, look, there's our dinner! Good, right on time.'

Whereupon Lia nudges me, winks and says: 'Oh well, another feast by the looks of it.'

I peer through the glass wall and see staff pushing two large aluminium serving trolleys.

Although I find some of Lia's jokes genuinely funny, the underlying problem is anything but. The more unhappy Muriëlle became during her stay at our nursing home, the more cynical she became. At first, if there was something she didn't agree with, she'd occasionally challenge the carers, but because she wasn't always taken seriously as a resident, I saw her become increasingly resigned to her situation. That said, like an old and battle-weary lion, she'll still have a go at someone from time to time. 'It's the only way I can show them what I'm made of, Teun,' she'll say, when she realises that I'm on to her. I really hope Muriëlle's move will go ahead, because a later life filled with cynicism is a very lonely life.

One by one, the plates are put down on the table, and the steaming, wobbling mass of beans settles. '*Bon appétit*, ladies,' I say and dig in, careful not to spill any. When I've polished off a second serving as well as trifle, a large filter coffee and a biscuit, I ask Lia: 'Fancy a walk?'

She practically jumps to her feet. 'That's an excellent idea!'

As we saunter up and down the corridors, she tells me about her colourful life as a musician and dancer in Amsterdam. 'I'm very well educated, you know. That makes it all the harder to end up in a place like this, where they only ever talk to you about the weather. I miss the depth that I had in my life, so I hope the two of us can bring some of it back.'

'Of course. My pleasure, ma'am. But would you mind telling me a bit more about your adventures in Amsterdam first?'

She takes my hand and gives it a firm squeeze. 'I'd love to. But if you really want to be my friend, you have to stop this ma'am business. I may be ninety-six, but that doesn't mean I act my age.' With that she gives me a wink and on she shuffles. I'm told that she used to trip the light fantastic at Paradiso, a well-known cultural centre in Amsterdam, and in the sixties she and her Hawaiian band used to tour with The Blue Diamonds. When we get to her room, she proudly shows me the pictures on the walls; they really bring her stories to life. 'See,' she teases me. 'And there you were, thinking that the old biddy was exaggerating?'

I pull a thumbtack out of the wall for a closer look at a black-and-white photo showing her at the age of around twenty, and I tease her right back. 'Well, I had to look twice to see if this was you. You look like a supermodel here.'

She appears to be on cloud nine. In one fluent motion, she performs a curtsey and gracefully throws her hair back, as if she's gracing the stage at Amsterdam's pop mecca again. '*Merci, mon amour...*' Before I have a chance to compliment her on her performance, her eyes take on a more strident look. 'See, that's exactly what I mean. During my time here, I've never had such a nice chat and so much fun as today.

Isn't that outrageous? Why they put me here in the first place, God knows.'

I move a bit closer. 'What do you think?'

She lowers her head. 'No idea. At the time they said: it's for your own good. But I liked it much better in my own home... I had friends and acquaintances nearby, unlike here.'

I find it nerve-racking to talk about such a painful topic, but I recognise both a need and an opening. 'So, how do you see the future? Because in four years' time you'll be 100,' I say, as Lia sits down on the edge of the bed.

'Pffff, I hope I don't live to see it. I've been here long enough. Let's face it, I'm no use to anyone anymore.'

Hunting for the right words, I say: 'Really, is that how you feel?'

'It's true, isn't it...? What's the point in me being alive?'

I'm trying to think of something to cheer Lia up, but I feel in everything that she means it. How is it possible that such a wonderful human being, someone with so many stories to tell, experiences her life in this way? And how sad must a person feel when death is a more attractive proposition? In an attempt to conclude the evening on a more positive note, I say: 'I'm certainly really pleased to have met you, and I hope we have many more wonderful conversations.'

She heaves a deep sigh. 'I hope so too, my boy, I hope so too... Off to bed you go. It's late.'

I give her a hug and cross the corridor to my room, where I collapse onto my bed and start crying. I'm shaken to my core. In the first eight hours of my visit here I've seen and heard so much sadness that I'm literally overflowing. I wish I could take Lia to Amsterdam so we can dance together till the early hours, walk along the canals while she's telling her wild tales and listen to music like there's no tomorrow. All to ensure that she doesn't experience the latter part of her life as a burden, but as something that does justice to who she is.

Three hours later I'm still staring at the suspended ceiling, so I decide to go for a wander round the unit to clear my head. It's not long before I realise that this isn't the best method to raise my spirits, because I'm greeted by a sight I only know from zombie films. I'm not saying this to shock or create bad blood, but because I'm bewildered by the nursing home's transformation after midnight.

It's as if some of the residents who'd been apathetic during the day have been revived yet can't see me. During the day, I saw Gerard sleep pretty much everywhere, but now he all but walks straight through me, as if I'm not here. Twice he approaches me like a stiff puppet with his eyes wide open, before literally bumping into me, standing perfectly still for a second and then shuffling back down the long, dark corridor.

I watch as Jannie, who spent the whole day rolling around in her wheelchair and only giggled a bit, talks to herself in full sentences in the bathroom mirror. 'Hey mum, good to see you again. Yes, it's me. I haven't seen Dad, but if that's how you're going to treat me, I'm leaving, you hear me?' She scrutinises her image in the mirror, as if she's trying to figure out who it is she's seeing. 'Right... Cheers then,' she resumes, picking up the medicine cup, filling it with water and raising it. I look on, mesmerised, while she's having this long imaginary conversation, and I'm beginning to understand why she's confusing the woman in the mirror with her mother. Dementia can sometimes take you back to earlier periods in your life; the grey hair and wrinkles she's seeing are incompatible with her self-image and remind her of her mother.

It's widely known that dementia can affect the circadian rhythm, but I've never seen it this bad. Everywhere I look, people are wandering the corridors, while others are sitting in pitch-dark living rooms staring wide-eyed into space. It makes me think that most of the residents are drugged up to their eyeballs with haloperidol, a classic antipsychotic that's still prescribed in nursing homes and causes these kinds of side effects. The following morning, my suspicion is confirmed. Gerard was given the medication when he became upset after suddenly finding all the doors locked to him. The staff had decided to put a stop to his snooping around in other people's rooms. His 'aggressive' behaviour was then deemed to be problematic and had to be 'flattened out' with haloperidol. Not only did it remove his curiosity and anger, but also his ability to recognise other living beings.

I genuinely wonder what's worse, the remedy or the disease. Why is a resident not allowed to open doors? What harm can he do when the rooms contain few if any personal items, let alone anything of value? Theft is impossible, as he can't take the loot anywhere. What else is he supposed to do? Spend all day sitting in a chair until lights out? What on earth do you do when you're not allowed to do anything? That's when you get wretched people who fly off the handle or who spend the whole day with their head slumped on the table?

The next morning I sit down to breakfast with what feels like mild jetlag from lack of sleep. I can tell Gon and Wil are waiting for me. 'Look, there he is. Did you sleep well, young man?' Gon asks.

While I help myself to two slices of soggy bread, a few pats of butter and a slice of cheese from the serving tray, I say:

'Like a baby!' The chair next to me remains empty, even when I'm halfway through my sandwich. 'Do you know where Lia is?'

'Oh, yes. She always has a lie-in,' Wil explains.

Gon adds: 'By the way, if you'd like coffee, it's behind you,' followed by a glance over my shoulder that leaves no doubt as to what she'd like me to do.

What a delightful pair, I think to myself.

'Let me get the thermos for another round of coffee.'

The ladies exchange satisfied glances.

On my way to the stainless-steel coffee trolley, where you can get your caffeine fix all day, I see the carers all drinking coffee together in the living room across from us and give them a friendly wave. It's a state of affairs that won't strike most people as odd, but ever since I started living in a nursing home it feels very stand-offish to me. A coffee break is traditionally a very sociable affair, a moment to enquire after everybody's wellbeing, but having it in two separate groups kind of undermines the homely atmosphere. It comes across as: right, that lot have had their coffee, now we can relax. Why don't the carers come and join us? Their stories about home or work are wonderful for people who don't have very eventful lives. And an added bonus: you don't have to be afraid of gossip spreading beyond the ward. Where to have coffee – it may seem insignificant, but it's details like this that can help create the sense of solidarity that so many people in this phase of their life crave. And the beauty is that these kinds of things can be changed overnight, without costing a penny extra.

Once I've served the ladies their coffee, I head over to the carers, because I'm curious to hear how they experience their workplace, and whether they feel the same as me. 'Good morning, everyone!' I exclaim to get us off to a good start. Initial conversations are usually a bit awkward, because I'm a kind of intruder who's been sanctioned by the 'boss'. Luckily, my questions are well-received, and it turns out that nobody would like to live here. But I also notice that few question why things are the way they are, or how they could be done differently. When the conversation turns to the changes that were introduced in the past, I sense a fair amount of frustration, which is articulated best by the lead carer: 'Every two or three years, another administrator comes along who wants to turn things round, but it's all just hot air. Before any of these changes are actually implemented, that person will have been promoted away, so everything stays the same.'

A harsh judgement, but it helps me understand the widespread reluctance to embrace change. Everybody has lost faith, so like Lia and Muriëlle the staff have become cynical about nursing homes. And when both sides have lost hope of a better life in care, it's no wonder that residents and employees alike become more and more frustrated. Somehow or other we need to rekindle hope.

Lia walks past, glances at Andre Rieu and says: 'That cheeky monkey again. Always scraping away on that violin of his.' At which she shuffles to the table and sits down.

Yup, I think to myself, that's it: we need hope!

And I walk to the living room to say hello to my new friend.

Two days later I'm in the centre of Beekbergen when I receive a phone call from Margje, who's interested to know how it's going. After I've brought her up to speed and I've told her that Lia is coming over to have a drink with me in the evening, she says: 'That sounds like fun, Teun. If there's a social gathering in my own nursing home, I want to be there.

So I suggest you buy an extra bottle!' I pop into a few shops to get some nibbles and conclude with a trip to the wine shop.

That evening I select Hawaiian music on Spotify, arrange the snacks on the table and light a candle. Then I cross the corridor and knock on my neighbour's door. 'Everything is set up, Lia. Are you ready?'

When I open the door a crack, I see she's applying lipstick. 'I'm keeping my pyjamas on, so I can crawl straight into bed later, but a touch of make-up is only right on an evening like this.'

While we're having our drinks, we talk about my life, my degree, love and we laugh at her saucy stories about the old days. I tell her: 'Tonight's my last night. How do you feel about the time I've spent here?'

Lia takes a sip of her red wine and thinks about it. 'Interesting, fun but also quite intimate, and that's what made it so special. If it were up to me, you'd be staying several more months.'

I give her a hug and that's when I notice Margje in the doorway, listening in on the conversation. We have another glass of wine together and then Lia announces: 'It's been a wonderful evening, dears. I've really missed this. I hope we can do it again soon, but I really need to go to sleep. *Bonne nuit!*' And with that she shuffles out of my room in her gold satin pyjamas and fluffy slippers.

'I love that you do this,' Margje says. 'It's weird how rare these things become once you're in my role, it's a real shame. So I won't be going home tonight; like you I'm staying overnight.' She raises her glass. 'Cheers. To more evenings like this!'

When we get onto my time at the home, she's amazed by what she hears, especially the bit about none of the staff wanting to live here. 'I understand where they're coming from, and I suspect that you feel the same after the past couple of days,' she says.

I nod.

'The place doesn't look very appealing, it's old, all of that's true. But if even we don't want to live here, then something's badly wrong. How can we make people feel that they've got a nice place here? That sense of homeliness is so important, and that's why I'm really glad you asked about it. We ought to start by creating a place or a home where we'd want to live ourselves, that would be a step in the right direction. The residents get to have a say in what they'd like, and it's up to us, the board, to figure out how to facilitate it. Change from the bottom-up, rather than the top-down, that's what we need. For that reason alone, having the two of you visit here has been priceless. It all begins with a small seed, and now that's been planted.'

I think about what the carers on the work floor told me. 'It's great that you're so open to it, but how are you going to help that seed grow? You've got an important role to play in that as an administrator.

She has a faint grin on her face when she replies: 'Excellent, that's the Teun I know. Actions speak louder than words. I spent years co-authoring the national policy and I know how hard it is to implement these things in practice. That's why I went back to working in the field. I firmly believe that we need to change the culture before a new policy has any chance of success. That's up to me, the board, the management, but especially the people on the ground. Let's not come up with yet another fad but work together to establish a new foundation. That's not something you can do overnight, but I do try my hardest every day.'

I pour another glass of red wine. 'That's the way I see it too. Everybody benefits from a pleasant culture, so let's start by making this a regular thing: drinks parties at the nursing home and good conversations. At mine next time?'

Margje laughs. 'It's a deal!'

III Europe's falling star

Care in Europe's poorest country

Moldova

Soon after we begin our descent, I spot immense Soviet-era blocks of flats through the window, surrounded by large tracts of green. It becomes clearer by the minute that we're about to enter a completely different world. That sense of otherness is reinforced by the spontaneous applause on landing, which suggests that flying isn't a common pastime here.

Wearing a colourful outfit and large vintage sunglasses, I walk into Chişinău Airport. I have a spring in my step. 'Man, I'm looking forward to this trip!' I shout to Jonathan, who's discreetly reorganising his camera bags. While still in the air, he started distributing his memory cards and hard discs across his luggage, because we were told that deep behind the former Iron Curtain, people aren't keen on prying eyes.

As we make our way towards border control in separate lines, I realise we're the sole foreigners. I'm not the only one to notice .... 'You, over there. This way!' a police officer says, waving his arm to tell me which way to go. When I look over my shoulder, I see that Jonathan is also plucked out of the queue. He towers over the three policemen, and his face says it all: here we go. Luckily, it turns out that he's not just a gifted film maker, but a pretty decent actor too, because in response to the barrage of questions he spins some tall tales about all those bags with camera equipment. He even tries to convince the small army of officers that the camera is not as big as it looks.

The word 'dementia' obviously doesn't mean anything to these uniforms, because the longer Jonathan goes on about the subject, the redder the faces of the otherwise pallid Moldovans become. Their patience is wearing thin and they're about to take us to an interrogation room when Jonathan holds up a document and shouts: 'Look, a letter from our government!' Bull's eye! 'Government' is clearly the magic word that defuses this heated situation. On hearing it, the officers calm down and a moment later they even help Jonathan carry his stuff.

He turns to me with a triumphant grin. 'See, Teun, it all works out in the end.'

When we're finally past border control, we see the relieved expression on our fixer's face. Marcella had warned us about a potentially rough landing. In the run-up to this trip, her input has been invaluable. Even though she's the head of a big school and mother to three children, she was on standby day and night, ready to help us navigate Moldovan bureaucracy as we tried to arrange our meetings.

When the terminal doors slide open, I feel as though I'm stepping forty years back in time. In the distance, I see brightly coloured but dilapidated buildings and enormous propaganda hoardings full of Russian symbols. Soon, my attention is drawn to a bunch of gigantic men in even bigger leather coats standing outside, eyeing us suspiciously from under their fur hats.

'Look,' Marcella exclaims, 'there's Pjotr. He'll be your driver.'

Another colossus of a man steps forward. He has a battered face full of scars that all but disappear when he flashes us one of the warmest smiles I have ever seen. He extends a huge hand and gently shakes ours and tells us in his best English: 'Hi guys, we're so pleased you're here. Come, let me take you to the hotel. You must be tired after travelling all this way.'

When Pjotr has put the suitcases in the boot and we get into the back of his sooty diesel Mercedes, I glance at Jonathan who, like me, is completely hyper after what we've just been through. As we drive off, he says: 'This is going to be special, I can feel it.' From the front, Pjotr says: 'Look, those are the Chişinău City Gates, also known as the gates of hell.' He looks over his shoulder and smiles. 'Welcome to Moldova.'

The republic of Moldova is in Eastern Europe and borders Romania to the west and Ukraine to the north, east and south. Until 1991, the country was part of the Soviet Union, and traces of that period still dominate the streets. Everywhere you look are big, grey blocks of flats from the Khrushchev era, when square footage was deemed more important than architectural design. As you go further into central Chişinău, you start seeing striking brutalist buildings, and it doesn't take a genius to figure out how the style got its name. With their geometric shapes, the massive concrete behemoths look more like monuments from the future than the past.

While these impressive edifices may suggest otherwise, Moldova is far and away the poorest country in Europe, and the government has made no provisions for dementia care.

This is exactly why we were so keen to come here. In our own country, more money is often seen as *the* key to better care, but is it really? And do people here see it the same way?

Pjotr weaves his way left and right through the narrowing streets, more and more slowly, until we come to a wide avenue and pull up outside a yellowish, castle-like hotel which looks like something out of a Wes Anderson film. With its clean lines in glass and concrete, it must have been an absolute gem in the Soviet Union's heyday – with the emphasis on 'have been'. Big red letters on the façade spell out a name that you wouldn't necessarily expect in this part of the world: MANHATTAN. But the current state of this once beautiful four-star hotel becomes all too clear when we look up at the entrance and see the fourth star dangling from the façade.

'Falling stars bring good luck,' I say as we walk through the big glass door and gently press the service bell at reception.

When we knock on Pjotr's car window at half four the following morning, we notice that he has moved his seat back and is fast asleep. I hope I'm wrong, but I get the impression that he spent the night in his car so as not to be late for our appointment. His old diesel has audible trouble starting and produces a plume of black smoke, but eventually Pjotr breathes a sigh of relief and tells us with his distinctive smile: 'I love German cars, they never break down.'

Ten minutes later, we collect Marcella at home and drive a long way out of the city. She tells us that our first location, a psychiatric hospital, is also the most challenging of our entire trip, because late last night the authorities told her that we might not be welcome anymore. On previous occasions, she'd already informed us that the government's intelligence services are still firing on all cylinders and very little escapes them, least of all foreigners wanting to take a peek behind the scenes. Since Moldova has no dedicated provisions for people with dementia, everyone with challenging behaviour and in need of round-the-clock care ends up in a psychiatric hospital. I'm incredibly curious to see how this works in practice, because I've never really understood why we group people with dementia together on the basis of their condition. Generally speaking, they are less responsive to stimuli, and this is exacerbated when they're all in the same place. Add to this the stimulus-free environment of a nursing home and the snooze fest is complete.

Suddenly, Pjotr slams on the brakes, and the two of us in the back are shaken about. It turns out that the road is full of enormous potholes that he has to drive around. Then we go through an old gate with faded lettering – we can just about make out the word PSYCHIATRIC – and the terrible road winds its way into a dense forest. It feels like a bad omen. That sense of foreboding only gets worse when we finally arrive at a car park where we're met by two men in long white coats.

Marcella gets out of the car to speak with them, and before long the three of them are engrossed in a discussion that we, despite not having any Romanian, can more or less follow because of the hand gestures. After thirty minutes of back-and-forth, a routine that's no longer entirely unfamiliar to us after the airport, Marcella returns to the car with good news and bad news. The bad news is that we're not allowed to visit the newer building on the site anymore. Last night, a government official phoned the director, the taller of the two men, and told him in no uncertain terms that he'd be sacked with immediate effect if he let us in.

Just then the man in question gestures for us to follow him.

'And what's the good news?' Jonathan asks as he shuts the door behind him.

Marcella gives the doctor a friendly nod, and as we follow the white coats she resumes. 'The good news is that we're allowed to visit the other houses. They've been empty since last week because they're awaiting repairs. That's why everyone has been temporarily moved to the building they don't want to show us. But this here is the place where people with dementia and other mental problems normally end up.' She points to one of the structures.

For a split second I think she's joking. 'No way, this one?' I say, staring at what I can only describe as a large World War II barracks. The filthy windows, most of which have been smashed, are fitted with steel bars.

Two more men, clearly security service staff, join us and the director says: 'You may go in now.'

The sound of the steel doors reverberates through the wide hospital corridors as we start our tour. Where daylight manages to penetrate the grimy windows, the darkness is illuminated by a greenish glow. At the first beam of light, I look left and see a white tiled room with small sprinkler heads attached to the high ceiling. Again, this reminds me of bygone war years, because it doesn't take a lot of imagination to understand that this is where people are collectively hosed down. The next room has five holes in the ground for residents to answer nature's call, and this is followed by a drab dining room and then, at the end of the corridor, the sleeping quarters.

'I can't believe it,' I say to Jonathan, as I walk past the steel beds with rubber mats. Without a thought for the somewhat nervous security officials, I well up. 'It looks like the residents have fled.' Items of clothing, hairbrushes and single slippers without their counterparts are scattered everywhere. The sickly scent of a life lived largely indoors is mixed with the pungent smell of urine, and a quick glance at the mattresses leaves no doubt as to where that stench comes from: they're covered in urine stains, both old and fresh by the looks of it. The azure wall panelling is covered in scratches and nicks, and my claustrophobia is complete when I realise that fifteen beds have been crammed into each room. 'What is this place?' I wonder out loud as I peer through the barred windows. 'This is inhuman, right? In the Netherlands many animals have a better life. How would...'

Bam! Bam! A few loud bangs jolt me from my thoughts. I look around and see that one of the security service guys is banging on the door and yelling: 'Enough, time to go!' His commanding tone leaves no room for debate. We exit the room and make our way back down the dark corridor but before we reach the exit we're overtaken by the echo of the unit door slamming shut behind us, and when we're all out the security guy locks the building with an old-fashioned passkey.

In the Netherlands we get worked up about the new coffee machine for the ward, the colour of the curtains or the prints to go on the walls, while people here can count themselves lucky with a bed and something to eat. Concepts such as quality of life, dignity, autonomy and person-centred care appear to be unheard of. Over here, living in a nursing home seems to be a matter of survival. The fact that we take so many things for granted in the Netherlands is rather humbling to me, but at the same time I wonder whether people really do live unhappier lives because of their living conditions. Or is that my own bias? I learnt early on not to project my own country's moral values onto other cultures. We may be used to flatscreens and spacious single rooms, but that's not to say that these also signify prosperity and wellbeing to people in other parts of the world.

A few days later we leave the capital Chişinău and head north. The gigantic Soviet blocks make way for fields as far as the eye can see, and horses and carts are starting to outnumber cars. As we drive deeper into the countryside, the landscape and the houses become more charming. Fruit trees and pastel-coloured fences brighten up the streets where children play and elderly people walk about at a pace that befits their age. Growing old here can't be too bad is the first thought that crosses my mind as we park the car, ready for our meeting with the Mayor of Greblești.

Precisely because the Moldovan government hasn't made any provisions for dementia care, I'm incredibly curious to see how people living with the condition are looked after in the community. Not least because the bulk of the population has no clear understanding of the disease.

At the town hall, which is no bigger than the small house next door, I'm met by a young woman in a bright yellow skirt. She greets me like her long-lost child. 'Teun, it's great to see you! Welcome to Greblești.'

After a brief pause – still somewhat taken aback by her trendy appearance in this old-fashioned setting – I respond with some Romanian words I learned on the flight, 'Er, thank you!'

Marcella has spoken at length with the mayor, Aliona Chricu, and asked her if she knows anyone locally who's dealing with the symptoms of dementia. Aliona knows everyone, so without a moment's hesitation she takes me by the hand and we head into the village. 'We have comparatively many older people here, because the younger generation has gone abroad, in search of a better life,' she says as she opens a pastel-green garden fence. 'This is Iulia's home, she's 93 and a lovely old dear. She lives here with her daughter, who does everything for her mother.'

The daughter seems a little shy but is clearly proud that we're visiting. Sitting in the garden, not far from a watchful dog that starts barking, I see an elderly lady hunched over her walking stick. Her floral headscarf makes the rural picture complete. We sit down next to her on the grass.

'Hello, ma'am, my name is Teun, and I think it's fantastic to see how you live here with your daugh...'

Before I can even finish my sentence, she starts talking: 'I'm really glad to be living at home and not at one of those places.' A statement she illustrates with a wave of her stick. 'That would be awful. Life here is good.' Despite the language barrier, I sense that she really means it.

I compliment the daughter on her dedication to and care for her mother, but when I turn to say goodbye old age has prevailed over the passionate resurgence earlier: the old woman has dozed off again. It makes her daughter laugh out loud.

'It's great to see you two so happy together,' I say. 'Long may it last.'

The woman nods, and after a hug we make our way further into the village.

As soon as we get to the next fence, I'm forced to change my idealised view of things. Ivan is in his late seventies and for some time now he has been living alone in a dilapidated farm. When we arrive, we see a few tea towels and trousers on a washing line and a well that gives an indication of the facilities that are available. Ivan's cognitive decline is making it harder and harder for him to look after himself, so he's wholly dependent on his neighbour, who's doing what he can to help with daily activities. Living at home is all very well, I think to myself, but you do need to have a support structure in place.

We hop onto a sprung cart with wooden spoked wheels, and when the boy on the box takes the reins we're off. To help me understand how people with dementia live at home, the mayor drops me off at Pastor Andrei Pirgaru, head of the local orthodox church and the community's social lynchpin. En route, the mayor explains that the pastor does home visits several times a week to see how people are doing and to hand them food that's been donated. 'A bit like Mother Teresa.'

When we get to the church, my stereotypical idea of a priest is turned upside-down, much like my image of a mayor earlier. A cool, youngish looking man with slicked-back hair in a cassock and a white clerical collar waves and as he comes striding towards us the large golden crucifix around his neck dangles back and forth. After handing the mayor a bag with things for someone in the village, he slaps the horse on its hind quarters. The animal trots off with my new friends.

'I'm really happy that you're joining me, Teun. People will be pleased,' the pastor says, as if introductions are an unnecessary luxury. He claps a hand on my shoulder and grabs my bag, and together we walk towards the immaculate white church with golden spires. Just like my mother when we have guests, our holy father apologies: 'Don't mind the mess, my friend...' At home, that's more out of politeness, but here we have to literally step over buckets of paint and dodge sticky plastic masking film before we get to his office. Everywhere you look are bin bags with blankets, cardboard boxes with hand soap and tins of food and stacks of round loaves.

'It may not be what you associate with a church,' Pastor Pirgaru says, 'but I try to help out where needed. We've been renovating the interior for years, and we really ought to use the collection money to buy new chairs, except that doesn't alleviate hunger, right?' And with that, he clamps as many loaves under his arm as he can, along with some nappies, and gestures for me to do the same.

Hugely impressed, I follow him to the field behind the church. As we head down to the lower-lying part of the village, I see gravestones sticking out of the tall grass on my left. Stray dogs bark viciously as we pass dilapidated barn-like cottages with lace curtains.

'Mind your head. The doorposts are very low round here,' the pastor says with a smile on his face, and tugs three times at a ramshackle door to get it to open.

Inside the damp little cottage, daylight filters through cracks, illuminating the icons on the wall. Lying on a bed is a squat little woman, covered in several knitted throws. It's clear that she's bunched them over her legs to hide something, and the minute we sit by her bedside the tears start flowing.

'You can't walk at all now?' the priest asks, cutting straight to the chase.

'I can't do anything anymore. I just lie here all day. They've even brought me a bedpan so I can relieve myself,' she says, and starts crying even harder.

'Oh, dear Elena, I wish I could do more for you. May God bless you and keep you, grant you patience and strength... The strength to carry on.' Pastor Pirgaru holds her hand a little longer, kisses it and leaves her some of the bread.

When I look back a final time, I see Elena through the window, waving at us, and it makes me appreciate all the more that if we want people to live at home for as long as possible, creating a good life for those with dementia is less a health-care matter than it is a social issue.

I've long thought that a decent standard of living is a basic human right, but in every house we visit I realise that it's a privilege. What choice do you have when life doesn't give you any options?

As mentioned, many younger folks have left, and it's becoming painfully clear what might happen to the older generations if the government fails to act. But when it comes to a better life is the government really *the* solution? We may be spending many billions of euros of taxpayers' money on care in the Netherlands, yet it doesn't seem to buy happiness for those in desperate need of it.

The stack of loaves under our arms is shrinking, and when we reach the final house on our round we walk straight into a Rembrandt painting. Through a delicate lace curtain, I look into a room where a very old lady in a floral dress and matching headscarf is sitting alone on a sofa. Slanting light from outside falls on her face and illuminates her gold teeth when she pops a boiled sweet into her mouth. Underneath her feet, which dangle against the sofa, a white kitten is playing with her leather flip-flops.

'Good afternoon, Alexandra, I've brought a visitor with me,' the pastor says as we enter. He sits down next to her, and as soon as he does so the little cat jumps onto his cassock.

The old woman laughs when he leaps to his feet in shock and his 'dress' blows up a bit. 'Welcome, Father, just stay where you are. My tiger is completely harmless.'

After serving us a glass of water, which is very refreshing after our walk, Alexandra starts sobbing too. 'I don't know how much longer I can go on like this, Father Andrei. What have I done to deserve this? I wish I had the Lord's blessing to go.'

The pastor throws me a glance in which I see more powerlessness than hope. 'My dear Alexandra, you're so brave. We can't determine our own fate, but I'll ask our Father in heaven to grant you your prayer.' Then he turns to me and starts talking. 'The church is the only organisation around here that looks after the old, because unfortunately the government doesn't care about the elderly. From the age of about sixty, older people in this country start feeling that they're a burden on society and would be better off put to sleep.' He falls silent for a moment, and I wipe the tears from Alexandra's cheeks. 'Thing is, Teun, all we have in life is the depth of our experiences. And when those fade, you have to have a pretty strong faith to remain hopeful.'

Moved by the visible fragility of life and the pastor's beautiful words, I give them both a hug when we part ways. How is it, I wonder, that our living conditions are so different, yet just like in Dutch nursing homes many people here would rather be dead than alive. When more money doesn't necessarily make a difference, I'd say there's something fundamentally wrong with the way we organise care for our elderly and vulnerable. Shouldn't we be focusing much more on what really matters and, where possible, facilitate that instead of creating 'a waiting room for death', as my friend Professor Anne-Mei put it so well?

Slightly dejected after everything we've seen, we go to meet our car the next day and find a surprisingly clean Mercedes. Pjotr is beaming. 'Today is a special day, guys...' He takes our bags from us and puts them in the boot. 'Because it's your final trip, I've given my "sweetheart" a proper polish.' We're fond of Pjotr, but we're pretty sure that our planned visit to the health minister played a role in his decision. During the past week, we've had to roll down the windows anytime we wanted to see something.

Pjotr drops us off at the parliament building in Chişinău, which is just as imposing as the presidential palace across the street. The Netherlands' own seat of government, the Binnenhof, is little more than a holiday cottage compared to the former headquarters of the once so mighty Communist Party. It's shaped like an upright open book, and positioned in the dead centre is an entrance flanked by four giant columns.

Once we've been screened and we've handed over our passports as security, I go to speak with the minister. I'm stunned to discover that one of the country's most powerful people barely even knows what dementia is. A lot of things fall into place now, but it also raises new questions. How do you deal with something that's unknown to you? And how can you look after a large group of people when you don't even know where to find them? Don't get me wrong: I didn't detect an ounce of disinterest or unwillingness on the minister's part. The man cares about people and is clearly moved by my words.

Many years of government corruption only served to make this country poorer, so to get Moldova back on its feet the emphasis had to be on economic recovery, the fight against poverty and basic healthcare. It's no surprise then that to date dementia hasn't been a priority. As the pastor explained to me, nothing will change as long as the population goes hungry. And shocking as the minister's lack of awareness may be, I do detect a sense of urgency in him that gives me reason to be hopeful. Not least because he'd like to meet again to learn more and plan for the future. To reinforce his words we pose, as is good practice, for an official portrait in front of the bright Moldovan tricolour. Then we continue on our way.

We have a long drive ahead of us. At the eleventh hour, Marcella has managed to locate a psychiatric hospital where we are allowed to meet people. This was high on our list after our experiences on day one and we don't want to miss this opportunity. The government normally complicates things, but the fact that the institution borders the 'breakaway and independent' part of Moldova may have helped secure this appointment. In the early nineties, this region, Transnistria, declared independence. During the brief civil war that followed the province received support from Russia's 14th Army, and their military might quickly put an end to the conflict. Although the Russian presence has been scaled back since, they still watch over Transnistria's independence, which has been recognised by few other countries. While the status quo continued, hostilities abated for a while, but at the time of writing, with the war between Russia and neighbouring Ukraine in full swing, the conflict has flared up again and Transnistria has seen an opportunity to bolster its secession.

After nearly three hours in the car, we arrive once more in a forested area with a psychiatric hospital. The exterior of the building, which looks like an old school, has metal cages attached to it, from which people are waving at us. It all looks so pleasant that to begin with I'm not sure whether these are covered balconies meant to protect people or whether they are supposed to stop them from escaping. When I come closer, I see a cage on the top floor with a group of older men who are smoking, and on the floor below lots of younger women who are curiously pressing their faces against the metal to get a better view of me. With these scenes reminding me of a prison, I'm apprehensive about what I might find inside. I make my way down the corridor and follow the arrows up the stairs, and at the top I'm met by a short man with a big moustache and the good old white coat. 'Hello, Teun. I'm Gheorghe, director and head doctor of this psychiatric hospital,' he says as he turns the key in a wooden door with glass panels. 'Come on in, I'll introduce you to our people.'

He gestures for me to go first and when I enter the ward I immediately feel all eyes on me. It's a large open space, bright and welcoming, with azure wall panelling and stylish curtains. To my left, I hear people cooking in a small kitchen just off the main room, but this sound is drowned out by giggling inside the room itself. It's getting louder by the minute, so I decide to sit down at a random table to see if I can connect with anyone. Women of all ages are slurping soup from tin bowls. Sitting across from me is an old woman in a red headscarf and a pearl necklace and crucifix over a blue-and-white striped dress. She calmly fixes her bright blue eyes on me and takes another spoonful of soup; she clearly has no intention of being distracted from her food. Her neighbour, a toothless young woman with facial hair, stares at me unashamedly.

'Hi,' I hear behind me.

I turn around and look into an even younger face framed by a funny bowl cut.

'I'm Teun. What's your name?' I ask.

When she smiles, I see that she too is missing most of her teeth. Without any hesitation, she gives me a big hug and says: 'I'm Nathalie. Where are you from?' She's still standing very close to me.

'Holland. Do you know it?'

She's quiet for a moment, then she frowns and shakes her head.

During our brief chat, about ten women have gathered

around us. When Nathalie hugs me a second time with the words, 'I like you,' they quickly form a queue after which Nathalie is shoved aside and the next candidate presents herself. Moved by this, I get to my feet, introduce myself and give her a hug. The line lengthens when the last few ladies join it. I was certainly not expecting this.

When I walk around the ward in the afternoon, the contrast couldn't be greater: I see people lying in dark rooms with multiple beds, where the ladies' entire wardrobes are draped over a single chair and the lino on the floor is held together with gaffer tape. But I also see lots of lively faces in the dining room, and I sense a solidarity here that I associate with a family setting. I see people wrapping their arms around each other and easy banter is followed by loud laughter. Younger women help older ones with their food, while others sing to each other, and in the corridor my new BFF Nathalie is comforting a woman who's sad.

How can it be that I'm seeing so many happy faces and such genuine concern for one another when these people get their fresh air in cages, sleep six to a room and have few if any facilities? I approach the director, who's watching the scene with a proud grin on his face, and tell him: 'I'm amazed by what I see. I can't think of any other location that has felt so inclusive right from the word go. What's your secret?'

He laughs, and then also gives me a big hug. 'As you can tell, we don't have a lot to show for, but we do have a lot to give. Our aim is to provide people with the best possible day; there must be room for everything, whether it's a sense of security or fun. I don't view these people as patients, but as my own children. I listen to them, compliment them, support them where I can, but above all I try to bring kindness to everything I do.'

Just when I thought I couldn't be more impressed.

'Nobody chooses to have the condition that brings them here, but as staff we have a choice in how to treat people. We can make sure that they like it here and feel safe. That's our objective.' And with that, the director makes his apologies, as he's needed on another ward.

He leaves me speechless. I can't get over the fact that within a day this country has given me back more than it has taken from me in a week. A few hours ago, I arrived here in very low spirits, but now I'm grinning from ear to ear.

This is what I'd been so keen to find: people of different ages and with different conditions collectively turning their facility into a real home. People opting for empathy, not apathy. And it's clear that this doesn't just make the residents happier, but the staff too.

When, at the end of the afternoon, a resident takes out her phone and puts on some folk music, the women take each other by the hand and start dancing. They soon notice that I haven't joined in, so Nathalie comes and pulls me into their circle. While swaying along to the music, I look at the radiant eyes of the women around me and I'm reminded of the falling star on the façade of our hotel. I can't think of a finer symbol for this trip and for this country.

IV The last pint

The end of an era

Utrecht, the Netherlands

'Fancy a cup of soup, Teun?' The question comes from the kitchen.

'Ooh, sounds good, Angelique. What kind of soup?' I reply and shut my laptop on the dining table.

'Let me check. I wasn't the one who made it... Chunky vegetable soup by the looks of it...' She stirs the pot with a big ladle and exclaims: '... with meatballs!'

Her enthusiasm makes me laugh. 'Great, just what I fancied.'

The housemates who were dozing at the table are beginning to stir, because of course they don't want to miss anything.

'I'll have a bowl too, please!' Tineke is the first to chime in, followed by the rest of the table in unison: 'Me too.'

I savour these moments, which you wouldn't normally experience in your twenties. You sense that in this home people live from meal to meal, and not just because of the fresh food we're served. There's always something going on around mealtimes. The kitchen staff liven up the place, while the smell of the food makes us feel good and gets everybody talking about favourite dishes. The atmosphere in the house is more relaxed, and the feeling that the walls are closing in on you is less acute.

When the plates are brought out we have a 'head count', just like my family used to have, so we immediately notice that someone is missing.

'Where's Elly?' I ask Ad.

'No idea, lad. I saw her in the corridor this morning, so she can't be far.'

The carers don't know either. I'm getting a bit worried, because rude as it may sound Elly is normally part of the furniture here. A while ago, her 'regular' wheelchair was replaced by an adapted tilt-in-space chair, which is what happens when your mobility deteriorates sharply. It's a clear sign of a new phase. As soon as the bread is served and everybody starts eating, I decide to go and have a look to see if Elly is all right.

It doesn't take me long to find her. When I step out of the living room, I see her standing in front of her room door. She's slumped against her wheelchair, hunched over and trembling.

I wrap an arm around her. 'Oh, dear Elly, what is it?'

'I-I-I...' she stutters and blubs. 'I'm really scared, Teun. Will you please stay with me?'

I press her close to me and say: 'Of course. Why are you scared?'

She rests her head against my chest and relaxes a little.

'I'm so scared that I'll be all alone when I go... You know what I mean? Will you please stay and hold me?' With that, she presses her head even tighter against me.

'Always, Elly, always...' I say, and gently stroke her hair. She's found herself in a few critical situations before, but each time she made a miraculous recovery. The big difference now is that she's lost a lot of weight, leaving her body far less resilient than it once was.

For most people, the prospect of the end is terrifying, so imagine what that must be like when you're no longer fully aware of what's going on around you and your experiences are now mostly internal ones. To me it evokes the idea of being locked inside a nightmare, from which it becomes harder and harder to wake up.

So it's perfectly understandable that Elly longs for a sense of security, even though she probably receives more visitors than anyone else on the unit. Her daughter Ellen is one of the warmest people I know, and it's heart-breaking to see the suffering caused by her mother's difficulties. When she visits Elly, she'll often come and have a coffee with me afterwards, and we've had some wonderful conversations. She really knows how to express what it feels like for a child and informal carer to go through something like this.

Only last week, Ellen told me how painful it is to bring your mother and best friend here, watch her become progressively more anxious and fearful and then leave her again after each visit. 'It's inhuman, Teun. I often beat myself up over bringing my mother here, but I didn't know what else to do,' she said with tears in her eyes. 'Surely, this isn't what the end of life should be like? Seriously, it may sound weird, but I love my mother so much that I'd be happy for her to go. I feel different about leaving since you moved in, because I know she'll get hugs and she has someone to turn to when she's afraid. But you're busy with school and all those cool initiatives to make the world a better place for people like my mother. And that's great, you know. Except... if that's taken away, then what's left? The carers here are all lovely people who help mum eat and drink, and that's all very well, but they don't seem to have the time for a nice one-on-one chat or a walk outside, which she loves so much. I really think there should be another way for us as a "civilised society".'

I could only agree and told Ellen about my experiences in Moldova: the degree of civilisation that I'd encountered over there could certainly not be measured by material wealth, care plans or the fanciness of the homes, but by the happiness of the people living in them instead.

'Tell the world what you're seeing and experiencing, and help bring about the change we need, Teun. Do it for my mother and all the others, okay?'

I made a solemn promise.

Meanwhile, Elly is half asleep in my arms. I whisper in her ear: 'Shall we have a bite to eat?'

She nods quietly, and I wheel her to the dining room, where the other housemates are already in front of the telly, in the grip of an after-dinner dip. 'Hey Angelique. I found her, but we had to have a bit of a catch-up. Is there any soup left, or has it all been hoovered up?' I ask.

'Oh, Teun, you know what it's like round here,' she says wryly. 'There's enough to feed an army. Sit yourselves down.'

I position Elly at the head of the table and take a seat on her right.

'Here you are, extra meatballs for Mr Toebes, and I've added a bit of cold water to Elly's soup so she can dig in straightaway. *Bon appétit*!' Angelique says as she wipes crumbs off the table.

'Thank you, you're an angel!' I say and immediately take a spoonful of my soup. It's boiling hot. That's what you get for only half-listening.

Journalists often ask me: 'Teun, what's changed in your nursing home since your book came out?' I understand the question, and I always respond in the same way: by stressing that I wasn't hired as some sort of change manager. I live here, and by talking about it I hope to initiate something; it's then up to the organisation to act on it. This may sound facile, but I'm afraid that's how it is. I can only identify the problem areas and potential solutions, but I can't enforce anything. By making my message as personal as possible, I try to appeal to the moral compass of those who are in a position to change things. And luckily, following the publication of my book, many of them have come forward.

Two of these people are the executives of the care organisation that runs the nursing home where I live. I've had a great relationship with Martin and Marie-Claire from the off. They've had total trust in me and have been really receptive to feedback. It takes guts for an organisation to be that open and vulnerable, and the fact that they've taken my criticism on board should be an example to other institutions. I've noticed that when the two of them decide to implement something, they immediately apply it to the organisation as a whole. It shows that change is possible. It really is. It may be a lengthy and difficult process, not unlike a large oil tanker changing direction, but that should never be an excuse to leave everything as it is. Besides, there are countless things you can do right now.

Take the fact that there are still trolleys with incontinence materials in the bathroom when I take a shower, that we're still not allowed to eat soft-boiled eggs and that the door to the enclosed garden is still locked. For me, as a resident, that's disappointing, all the more so because I know that these are things we could change today. We seem to have become so bogged down in the processes of committees, interest groups and other organisations that any improvements are slowed down, or perhaps we just don't feel the urgency. But if we don't take action now, this can be our own future.

Another problem is that many commercial care providers see nursing home care as a goldmine and try to keep generating income by leaving everything as it is. This means that all the classic safety and control mechanisms for residents are constantly repackaged in expensive new technologies and innovations. From a commercial perspective this makes a lot of sense, given that the 'freedom model' isn't a big money-spinner.

Take the 'leefcirkel', for example, literally living circle, but this technology is sometimes translated as 'degrees of freedom', but I think of it as 'locked door 2.0'. It's supposed to give residents more liberty, but it really only moves the problem of confinement elsewhere. For our house alone, the price tag for the system, which my housemate Wil aptly refers to as 'the modern ankle tag for people with dementia', is just shy of 200,000 euros, and that's not counting the annual maintenance costs. The official definition is as follows: 'a "leefcirkel" is a care technology for people with dementia. A resident is fitted with a tag that "customises" their freedom of movement. Some doors open for them, others remain locked.' In practice this means that many residents still end up standing in front of closed doors and see that some are allowed 'out' while others are not. Try and explain that! Those who are allowed to go through the first door will then be knocking fretfully on the next, because they don't understand why some open and others don't. 'I thought I was allowed out?' And the rare individual who gets to go even further has to be monitored by the carers, like some sort of 'track-and-trace parcel', to make sure they don't go anywhere that's off-limits.

In short: there's still no freedom for residents and even more pressure on an already expensive care system. It's the opposite of what we want to achieve, if you ask me. To create *real* solutions, we need the courage to have other conversations and accept that nursing homes are not places where we can put people safely behind lock and key. A real home is for living, with risks such as falling over, bumping into things, choking on food, not wanting to eat from time to time and feeling angry and sad – just like you would at home.

That's one of the reasons why I'm so keen to visit places that are already working in this way, whether it's a recent or a more established practice, to show people that we can do things differently. Seeing is believing is as true in the care sector as it is in other walks of life.

So trust me… we'll get there.

From my blue vintage sofa by the window, I look out at the first tentative signs of spring. Normally, I find it the most joyful time of the year – animals give birth to their young, the sun grows stronger and the trees boast gorgeous shades of fresh greenery – but I've been feeling sombre for days now. Even my housemates have noticed. 'You're very quiet, Teun,' Ad said to me this morning. 'If you need help, you'll tell me, right?' If there's one thing I'm terrible at, it's pretending, yet I responded with a fleeting smile: 'Of course, Ad. I think it's just my seasonal dip lasting a bit longer than usual…' Meanwhile the knot in my stomach grew bigger and bigger.

A week ago, after much umming and ahhing, I decided to leave the home I've lived in for two years. I haven't told anyone yet. However well I've been treated here and however much support I've received from the organisation, I can't help but feel a heavy weight on my shoulders every time I enter the unit. On the other side of the locked doors, I can talk passionately about my mission to improve conditions for people with dementia, but in here I'm often on the brink of tears. I'm tired after everything that's happened; fed up with the day-to-day tension, the constant battle to encourage debate, the heartache that lurks everywhere.

Saying goodbye to Eugenie, a few weeks ago, was the final straw for me. The woman had been a ray of sunshine in our home from the very beginning. She never put herself centre stage but was always available for an encouraging glance and a nice chat. I could sit beside her for hours without a word and still walk away feeling content. She was easy-going and broad-minded, and that felt exactly right. When she told us that she was very poorly and that we'd better say our goodbyes, something inside me snapped. In the past two years I'd watched many housemates 'cross over', but this time I couldn't handle it.

Sobbing, I followed Ad to her room, where the blue afternoon light coming through the net curtains seemed to reinforce that cold permanence of a final goodbye. Eugenie was lying in bed; she looked serene but was no longer responsive. My friend grabbed a folding chair and sat down, distraught, and did something he'd never done before. He took my hand, squeezed it tight and said: 'Go ahead, lad, have a good cry.' We sat there, hand in hand, without talking, just like we used to do with Eugenie. And again, for the very last time, it felt exactly right.

For a few days, I barely left my room, which gave me the chance – in the middle of a hectic period – to finally reflect on everything that had happened and what I wanted to do next. Something had to change, that much was clear. Earlier,

I'd been determined that after leaving the nursing home I'd live a 'normal' life in student digs, but I was having second thoughts. Instead, I decided to go to another nursing home, this one in Amstelveen, just south of Amsterdam. It began to dawn on me that I wasn't necessarily trying to escape this way of life, but the intensity of the experience. For the nursing home, the organisation and myself, this style of communal living was uncharted territory, so these past few years I've felt as if I've been living inside a pressure cooker. And now the pressure had literally become too much. To ease it, there was only one thing I could do.

Feeling as if I'm about to break up with a partner, I finish my coffee, look in the mirror and tell myself: 'You can do it!' Then I spritz on some aftershave, pull the door shut behind me and head over to the organisation's headquarters where I have an appointment with the board of directors.

My nerves all but dissolve when I find them very understanding of the 'separation' and they promise me their continued support for my mission, albeit from a distance. Martin, one of the executives, concludes our meeting with some kind words: 'You taught us to listen even better to our residents, Teun, and you really held up a mirror to us. For this, we thank you.' Then we shake hands and say goodbye.

On my way back to the unit, my feet grow heavier with each step closer to the 'real divorce' awaiting me. The first room on the left behind the closed door is Ad's. I've decided not to lie to my best friend here and to give it to him straight, so I knock and say: 'Ad, are you home?' When I carefully stick my head round the door, I see him.

'Where else would I be?'

I laugh. That's the kind of remark I needed as an icebreaker. 'I won't beat about the bush, mate, although I'm nervous about telling you this, but... I'm leaving.'

Ad looks at me approvingly. 'Oh, I knew you were, lad. I'm not surprised, this is no place for a twenty-year-old! I'm going to miss you, but you should go. Just promise me one thing: don't forget me, will you, kiddo?'

I breathe a sigh of relief, and I'm overcome by a sense of melancholy. 'Ad van Dokkum,' I begin. I never use his full name, so he knows I really mean it. 'Do you really think I'd leave and forget all about you? Never, Ad! I'll keep visiting, whether you like it or not.'

With a big grin on his face, he says: 'Excellent, looks like we have a deal.'

Not much later I'm in my room, and when I take a final look around I think: this is it, then, the end of the two most remarkable years of my life. Then I put together the first moving box and take my 1980s records off the walls, my books off the shelves and the disco ball off the system ceiling. About ten boxes later, I'm ready to pack the floral French dinnerware my mother gave me. As I make a start, with some great techno music on my AirPods, I hear a gentle knocking. It soon grows louder.

'Hey, are you deaf, or what? Take those hearing aids out!'

When I look over my shoulder, I see Ad and Tineke in the doorway. Completely taken aback, I remove my earphones and exclaim: 'Ah, have you come to help? That's so sweet!'

Ad manoeuvres Tineke's wheelchair deftly past the boxes and parks it next to my sofa. 'No, I don't think so. You've got so much clutter.' He looks around in astonishment. 'We've brought a nice cake to thank you for our wonderful time together.'

I swallow hard to stop myself from getting emotional; saying goodbye may well be the hardest thing to do. 'Wow, that's so incredibly sweet of you.' I lift a couple of boxes off the sofa, so Ad can sit down. 'Right, if you sit over there, we all just about fit. How about a coffee then?'

I think that many people won't believe me when I tell them that my housemates with dementia surprised me on my final day at the nursing home. If I had a penny for every time someone joked to me: 'Luckily your housemates will forget that you ever lived there.' Or: 'After a week they'll no longer know who you are, so I wouldn't worry too much about that move.' Sure, sometimes they forget events and situations, that's true. But if I've been elsewhere for a week, Ad always demands to know why I've been away so long and he's curious to hear what I've been up to. Of course, that's not true for everybody here, but it's wrong to assume that nobody remembers anything.

'Will you come and have a beer with me this evening, for old times' sake?' I hear from the sofa, and I see that Ad and Tineke are digging into their second piece of cake.

'I'd love to. But only if you help me carry these in a minute.'

Ad looks up in shock with his mouth full of cream and says: 'Yes, I thought as much.'

At the close of day, my housemates sit on their walking frames right by the fence, watching me fill the removal van to the brim. After closing the tailgate, I receive a smattering of applause from the removal jury.

'That's it,' says Juul, and gives me a thumbs-up.

'You're not rid of me that easily,' I tease her as I open the car door. 'I'm only taking my things to Amstelveen. I'll be back to say goodbye, OK?'

After seeing more thumbs up, I hoist myself behind the

wheel, turn the key and round the corner, all the while pressing the horn. It really takes me back. Exactly two years ago, I also drove along the Amsterdam-Rhine Canal with a van full of things, but with this difference: I've now gained a world of experience.

It's already dark when I get back, tired from all the lifting, and key in the code for the last time, 2-0-1-7. Once I'm on the ward, I turn left to go to Ad's room. 'Did you get the beers in, Ad?'

From the big armchair in which he's watching a random football game he yells back: 'What do you think? The fridge is chock full.'

When I open the small fridge, I see that we have some specialty beers to look forward to. 'This is going to be quite the farewell party. Yum! I'm going to give the others a hug and then I'll join you, OK?'

Because it took me a while to unload the van, I'm back later than I'd hoped and most of my housemates are already in bed. Luckily, the light's on in Tineke's room, so I quickly make my way over. When I push the door ajar and see that her eyes are still open, I give her a goodnight kiss and whisper in her ear: 'I'll be back soon, dear Tineke, promise.' She presses her cheek to my face and lets out a contented sigh.

After a final inspection of my room and a hello to the nightshift, I flop down on the chair beside Ad. I'm on my last legs. 'Oof, I've never been more ready for a beer.' That's when I notice that Ad has already taken two out. 'You're the best, Ad!' I say, and we clink our bottles together.

'I'll be honest with you: I'm going to miss you, kiddo.' Ad looks at me, not sure what to say next. He raises his eyebrows.

'Yes, same here, Ad. A lot.' Again, I clink my bottle against his. 'You've become a really good mate, and the great thing is, good friends last forever. We're going to do plenty more fun things together.'

I can tell he's struggling to wrap his head around all this, so I keep quiet for a bit.

We sit staring at a TV match between two clubs from some faraway football league, and after a while he says: 'I know you won't forget me and that things are going to be different for me from now on... but I'm glad we became friends, I really am. When I first moved here, I was tired of living. You know that. But when you joined us, I was reminded of how much fun life can be. With you I didn't feel like a sick old man, with you I went out and about. We rode a motorbike together, had fun in the pub, watched football, while I talked about love, sex and beautiful women. I actually felt happy at times, and that was something I never thought I'd experience again. For that I want to thank you.' He picks up his bottle. 'To you!'

I respond with tears in my eyes: 'To us, my friend, to us!'

When Ad takes a sip, he realises that he's already finished his bottle. We both laugh.

'Give me that,' I say and get to my feet. 'You can't propose a toast with an empty bottle, certainly not after such fine words. Come, let me get the last beer.'

V Glazed over

The beginnings of another perspective on care

Denmark

Anyone driving through this landscape can't help but feel at peace: undulating green pastures form a sharp contrast with the clear blue sky and sea, and bright yellow rapeseed fields unfurl when we round a hill. A privileged place on earth, it feels like. A little later, the built-up world comes into view again, with colourful fisherman's cottages and whitewashed farms with thatched roofs – again, fabulous – but as soon as Jonathan turns left into a car park, the magic evaporates.

The drab, low brick building, which appears to date back to the 1980s, raises certain expectations that are quickly confirmed on entering: the musty odours of overcooked cauliflower and laundry trolleys crowd out the fresh sea breeze. Am I going to find this country identical to my own, I wonder, as I quietly wheel my suitcases across the familiar lino.

If there's one region that's said to have the best care in the world, aside from the Netherlands, it must be Scandinavia. The Scandinavian countries are placed high on nearly every list containing the word 'quality' and are seen as the standard bearers for a long and happy life. The large sums of money that are invested in healthcare usually get a mention too, but that's not the reason why nearly all the researchers in our preliminary study referred to Scandinavia as the future of dementia care. So to find out whether the grass really is greener in the north, we'll be taking an in-depth look at this 'cradle of happiness', starting in Denmark.

After we've decided who gets which bed, I've chucked my clothes into the wardrobe and Jonathan has taken out his camera, we make our way to the living room, where we find a cup of coffee waiting for us with what looks like a homemade biscuit.

I'm pleasantly surprised to find that this home has comparatively many men and therefore a nice mixed crowd. 'Hmm, that looks good,' I say as I sit down next to a man wearing a red cap and bite into my cookie.

He gives me a friendly nod, but clearly can't quite place me.

The woman opposite me is more outgoing and immediately starts talking to me in English: 'I bet you're not from here. Are you from France, by any chance? You look French with those luscious curls.'

I smile and tell her that I'm from the Netherlands.

'Really?' she asks. 'I would never have guessed, and I should know, because I've seen half the world.' Over the top of her pink designer specs, which rest on the tip of her nose, she looks at me as if to say: I'm not kidding.

'I'm envious,' I reply enthusiastically, and in an attempt to continue the conversation I add, 'My name is Teun. What's yours?'

Again, she looks over her glasses. 'Hm, now you mention it, that does sound very Dutch. But those curls...'

A carer who's been listening in at the head of the table joins the conversation with a smile on her face. 'Our diva

Kate isn't easily persuaded. He only just got here and you're already teasing him, Kate?'

Kate decides to show her who's boss. 'Sorry, I don't know what you're talking about, but this young man and I were having an interesting conversation. Isn't that right?' I can tell by the look on her face that I'd better answer in the affirmative.

This is great, I think to myself, and take another sip of my coffee. Perhaps this place doesn't embody the big change I'd hoped for, but the people who live here are already making this visit special. And the location adds to that feeling, because I haven't seen any other nursing home that's right by the sea, overlooking a gorgeous coastline with white beaches.

When the sun climbs above the tall fir trees beyond the fence and the afternoon gets underway, I see residents going outside to warm themselves in the rocking chairs. Look at that, I think, so this is what happens when you open the door to the garden: people come to life. None of that staying indoors, like we do in our country, where jugs of water and ice lollies are meant to combat the heat. It's much nicer to go out and feel the wind in your face, take a nap in the sun or go for a refreshing walk under the trees. An open patio door may seem like a small thing, but it makes a huge difference. The world you live in becomes literally twice as big. These kinds of experiences can make the final stages of life so much more bearable and, who knows, maybe even give it some meaning.

It's a good first step towards a better quality of life, but while the surroundings here may be idyllic and the people treated lovingly, their freedom still doesn't extend beyond the fence. A painful illustration of this follows a little later when I'm out for a stroll with Kate. As we walk down a gravel path past beautiful wild flower beds and pick up where we left off this morning, she suddenly says: 'Do you happen to know the code to the lock?'

The question catches me off guard, even though I know exactly what she means. I reply in as neutral a voice as I can muster: 'What lock?'

Kate looks at me as if I'm playing her for a fool. 'Of the fence, of course!'

This beautiful garden is enclosed by a large, green steel fence, which detracts from the even more beautiful sea view. Kate tugs at it and fidgets with the combination lock, and as I look on a little uneasily she starts to panic. 'I want, I want...' she says in a shaky voice, before suddenly screaming at the top of her lungs: 'I want out! I want... out!' She yanks even harder and yells: 'Let me out!'

I wrap an arm around her and say: 'I don't know the combination either, honestly.'

She fixes those pleading eyes on me again, as if she's trying to gauge whether I'm pulling her leg. 'Well, how could you? But I can't wait to get away from this place. They know that, but they won't let me out.'

Kate lets go of the fence, and we continue our walk.

The incident hasn't gone unnoticed by the staff, including manager Mette Sophie, who comes over to warmly greet Jonathan and myself. 'Welcome, it's so nice to have you!' But then her face clouds over. 'I do hope you won't just use this bit for the film?'

We both give her a hug, and I say: 'We'd never show just one thing, because we're keen to learn from the countries we visit. But this is part of the world here, isn't it? I'd say this was a learning opportunity too.'

Mette thaws at once. 'True. It's just frustrating, because

we're trying so hard to create a great place where people with dementia can be happy, with freshly cooked food every day, a nice garden and the kind of loving care that gives everyone as much freedom as possible. But yeah...' She heaves a deep sigh. 'We have our vision, but that ugly fence remains a thorn in our side. The local authorities won't allow us to remove it, because they're afraid our residents might come to harm. I can't really tell Kate to take the issue up with the council. We have to work within the regulations, which is difficult at moments like this. But not trying to do the best job possible isn't an option, is it?'

This is exactly why we rated Mette so highly during our research phase in the Netherlands. We got to know her through Anneke Draper, a Dutch care assistant and acquaintance of mine who'd moved to Denmark. She told us about this 'formidable and energetic administrator who sees opportunities everywhere to improve care and who makes decisions from the heart.' This sounded like the ideal first stop in Scandinavia to us, something that was confirmed during our subsequent conversations with Mette.

Because she doesn't just say the right thing at expensive conferences and seminars but is always trying to implement her vision on the ground, I understand her sense of frustration only too well: while there's a will to change, there's not yet a way.

'I'll leave you to look around and get a sense of the place,' Mette wraps things up. 'I need to check whether my husband hasn't drowned. He went on a long canoe trip around the Isefjord.' She winks at me and when she gets to the door, she turns round one last time. 'Oh, before I forget, I hope you two are coming for a swim with me tomorrow morning?'

'Oh no, I forgot to bring my swimming trunks!' I say.

Mette looks surprised, but then she smiles. 'No problem, we don't wear them here.' And with that she walks out into the corridor where she shouts: 'See you tomorrow, guys!'

Meanwhile the table has been set, and I take a seat next to this morning's neighbour, Anders with the red cap. He appears to have a bit more faith in me, because this time I'm not greeted with a nod but with a friendly 'hello'. As I tuck into the fresh fish that's so beautifully arranged on my plate, I can't stop thinking about this one question: when care is so well-organised from the top down, and there are cheerful carers who treat people with love and you're free to wander into the garden, why do I still feel that I wouldn't want to live here myself? It's not a criticism, more a sensation that sometimes comes over me barely five minutes after walking into a place and that doesn't go away in the hours or days that follow.

Because we spend long hours on the road and we're constantly thinking about what we're seeing, why we're seeing it and what it might mean, it's usually late by the time everything's been uploaded and downloaded and the camera is packed up again. On the one hand it's pretty tiring, but it also gives us a glimpse into a world we wouldn't see at an earlier time.

While Jonathan is downloading the most recent footage onto his computer, I open our exterior door and ask over my shoulder: 'Fancy a beer?'

'Yes, please. I'll be right there.'

What a joy it is after a long day to let go of all the stress with a beer out on the patio, I think to myself as I gaze up at the remarkably clear starry sky. Just as I pull open my can with a loud hiss, I see some frantic movement behind a window across from me. It's Kate. She signals that she's pleased to see me and is coming out too, followed by equally frenetic gestures suggesting that under no circumstances should I go back inside. She's the only one round here who'd be as naughty as that, I reckon, while I take a sip of my beer and give her a thumbs up to say that I'll wait.

Every room has its own little patio measuring five by five tiles surrounded by beech hedging that appears to be high enough to discourage people from climbing over. Then again... no hedge stops the truly determined. Kate opens her door and clambers over it. 'Right, what shall we do?'

Meanwhile, Jonathan has also joined us outside with a beer, and we have to do our best not to laugh too hard, because we can tell that she's dead serious. 'Eh, what do you mean by, "What shall we do?"' I feign naivety.

'Well, I like a party, so I thought: I'm going out with my new friends. Somewhere, anywhere, I don't mind. So, what shall we do, gentlemen?'

Like in a scene from the film *Untouchable*, I can picture us escaping to the local pub and coming back blind drunk, but I realise that we'd never get Kate home again if we did that. Maybe that's part of her plan, because if there's one person who has shown us right from the word go how cunning she is, it's our opposite neighbour, who's now munching our crisps.

So I wisely say: 'It's our first night here, so we're staying in, if that's OK with you?'

The spontaneous al fresco drinks appear to have tempered her wild plans a little, and she looks happy enough with the situation. 'Good idea.'

We chat about her global adventures and the places she'd still like to visit, and very late at night I walk her back to her room, tuck her into bed and switch off the light. 'Sleep well and see you in the morning, Kate.'

'Bye, lad,' I hear from the bed.

'What a wonderful woman,' I mutter to myself as I clamber back over our hedge. In our room, Jonathan is already out for the count, and as I'm drifting into dreamland myself, my last thought is: what a day!

After a few hours' sleep, we're woken up by two iPhone alarms going off. Swimming at five in the morning. Whose idea was that? I quickly throw on a warm jumper and take a towel from the bathroom.

Still half asleep, we accept Mette's lift to the harbour, where we see that she isn't the only Dane to have risen at this hour. 'We're not doing this because you're here, we do this every day. It's part of our culture, a refreshing start to the day in the water that surrounds us,' Mette explains as I see a group of people in bathrobes walking up the jetty, young and old alike. For some reason, I thought this was going to be a fun little swim outing – my knowledge of geography and climate leaves something to be desired – but Mette is quick to dispel that misunderstanding: 'the water's around five degrees Celsius, so really cold, but that's why it's so good.'

I'm in shock after 'five degrees', so barely even hear the word 'good'. And as if that isn't bad enough, she says: 'Kit off and in we go.'

As though this is an everyday thing for me, I drop my boxer shorts and step into the ice-cold water, right behind a naked nursing home manager I first met yesterday.

A little later, with our 'Danish baptism' behind us, we sit down to a breakfast of yoghurt, fresh fruit and delicious oatmeal cookies that I can't get enough of. I'm about to take a sip of orange juice when my neighbour, who's wearing a different colour cap today, actually asks me a question: 'Good morning, lad, did you enjoy your swim?'

I put down my glass. 'Absolutely, but you Danes are mad to be jumping naked into an icy sea every day.'

Anders clearly doesn't take it too personally and bursts out laughing; I appear to have passed my integration exam. Really connecting with someone is the best feeling there is, I think to myself, and take another bite of my oatmeal cookie.

That morning I get to witness Mette's approach in practice. While the weekly Elvis impersonator is playing live music, the staff are lovingly taking the residents by the hand for a spin. Even the wheelchair users are given a gentle twirl. When I decide to pop to the toilet in between renditions of 'Jailhouse Rock' and 'In the Ghetto', I'm shocked to find one of residents flat on the floor. I run over to see if anything is wrong, but Frida is just lying there, staring into nothingness, totally relaxed. Upon arrival, I was told that she's no longer verbal, so to verify my assessment, I walk over to the nearest carer, who's also dancing.

'Excuse me, I noticed that Frida's on the floor. And...'

Before I can even finish my sentence, the carer says: 'Oh, she always does that. She really enjoys the underfloor heating, and while it may look weird we want her to be happy. So don't worry about it!' She turns around and carries on dancing.

Wow, that's remarkable, I think on my way back to the toilet. This must be one of the most striking examples of person-oriented care that I've come across. Checking to see what the resident needs and accommodating it, however strange it may look to people without dementia.

After my pitstop, I sit beside Frida on the floor for a while and I begin to understand why this place still feels like an institution, however warm and cosy it is: like in the Netherlands, much of the cosiness and liveliness is generated by staff and through external stimulation. As soon as the meals, the coffee breaks in the sun and other activities are over, most of the residents here withdraw into their own world because they're no longer stimulated. And so they too stare into space all day.

In Moldova I didn't once feel that people had to be entertained with food, an Elvis impersonator or a craft club in order to be happy. Personal interaction was enough. How come people in the Western European homes I've visited all display that typical 'apathetic' behaviour and are incapable of keeping themselves occupied? It's not the surroundings – I've never seen a nursing home in such a prime location, with a sea view to boot – and it's not the cordiality of the staff, let alone Mette's vision. But all these things still don't make this nursing home a real home. I can certainly identify efforts to improve the quality of life here, but I feel as if there's something essential missing, something that allows people to really *live*.

From the corner of my eye, I see Kate heading in my direction. Very, very slowly, she shuffles across the floor, the same floor on which her gaze is fixed. Very odd. No 'friend' this and 'friend' that, like before, and no witty remarks about my appearance. None of that.

I approach her and ask if she'd like to have a coffee with me. There's little or no reaction. As I escort her to a rocking chair outside, I notice that she's very confused and can barely string a sentence together. This isn't the Kate I know, I think when I go to fetch two cuppas.

Back inside I ask what's going on and I'm told that after our chat Kate tried to escape a few more times by forcing the main door with a broom stick. In consultation with her family, it was decided that, 'if necessary', she could be given some calming medication. Her spark, her wry wit, her wild tales and her mischievousness – they're all gone. Escaping is not only physically impossible now, but mentally too.

I ask Mette if I'm allowed to take Kate to the sea, which she loves to gaze out at, to see if that will cheer her up. It's allowed. I grab a warm coat for Kate and a bottle of rosé from my suitcase, and arm in arm we exit via the side door, walk halfway around the house and end up on the 'right' side of the fence on the beach. These are the kinds of moments when Mother Nature likes to lend a hand, and sure enough, she has produced another beautiful sunset. The smooth sea reflects the purplish-red sky like a mirror, swans are swimming towards the horizon and the sun is so big we can almost touch it. I kneel to lay down my coat and to plant the bottle of wine in the loose sand, and then realise how romantic this must look from a distance.

'Don't you think this would be the perfect moment to propose to you, Kate?' I flash her a smile. 'You'd say yes, wouldn't you?'

For a split second we have contact: she nods. But immediately after, her eyes glaze over again.

We sit down on my coat, and she leans into me while the sun changes colour. 'Isn't that beautiful?' I say with my arm around her.

I hear a very soft 'beautiful.'

A few days later we thank Mette for her hospitality and the unforgettable experience and head northwards across Denmark's biggest island, Zealand. The land of the Vikings consists of two parts, which were united in the tenth century BC by King Harald Bluetooth. The 'mainland' in the west, Jutland, borders Germany and is characterised by rough seascapes and forests. The eastern part consists of an archipelago of no fewer than 444 named islands, many of which are inhabited. And while Zealand's coastline may be rugged and steep, the interior landscape is undulating and gentle, so that within the space of an hour we find ourselves in a totally different world. Eventually, we stop outside a red farm-like building.

A brown golden retriever comes bounding towards us as we take our suitcases out of the boot. In the distance, we hear the bleating of goats. It's quite the welcome, I think to myself as we enter the house. At the long table in the dining room, someone with headphones on is listening to music; she glances at me, waves and never stops swaying her upper body to the rhythm of what must be pretty catchy tunes. To my right a woman with long silvery grey hair is helping a man in a wheelchair, probably her husband, drink something. As I'm scratching my head about the peculiar chairs at the back of the room, two young women in smart pale blue shirts walk in.

'Good morning,' one of them says. 'Please take a seat and make yourselves comfortable. Did you find the place okay?'

No sooner do we sit down than we're served coffee and cake, and I answer: 'Yes, but it would have been a totally different story without GPS.'

The women nod, sit down as well and introduce themselves. I'd already recognised founder May from our Zoom calls. She's pleased to see us, she says, and is sure we'll feel at home here. 'You can do as you please, but we do ask you to be quiet in that corner over there. That's where the massage chairs are for people to relax in.'

Ah, so that's what they are. 'I take it we're allowed to sit in them as well?' I ask, whereupon everybody bursts out laughing.

'As you can probably see,' May continues, 'we go for an authentic environment here with real things. We get fresh flowers delivered every week, cook three fresh meals a day and in the evening we light candles to create a cosy atmosphere. As I always tell my staff, if we have the courage to burn candles, we're on the right track. That means we have the courage to trust people and make this a real home.' She smiles. 'And the beauty is that nobody has burnt themselves in the past few years and the house is still standing.

The woman sitting across from us at the table chuckles at this and makes no attempt to hide that she's eavesdropping.

It's as strong an introduction as they come, and I've already heard things that would be inconceivable in other places. Real candles? Right here on the table? In my country, they don't even trust people with real plants, let alone with something that might cause actual damage. Then again, there might not be any point to candles in my home, as the overhead lighting is always on and ruins any chance of cosiness.

It's certainly very different here. I see beautiful floor and table lamps, chandeliers and even some reading lights beside the sofa, and it's weird to think that I find that extraordinary. The walls here don't have stock photos with kitschy quotes, antiquated landscape paintings or saccharine animal prints. No, there are real paintings here, by real artists, behind real glass. And everywhere there are beautiful plants in even more beautiful pots and flowers in vases. For the longest time I've been trying to explain the difference between a house and a home, and my ideas are often dismissed as idealistic and unattainable. But this place illustrates just how incredibly easy it is to take the first few steps towards achieving that. Do we really think it makes more sense to spend over 20,000 euros on fake plants, as they did at a nursing home I visited recently, than to create a genuinely homely feel for a handful of euros?

After we finish our coffee and cake, we make our way to the basement, where we get to spend the night in the meeting room. We prefer not to take up space meant for residents, so it's always a bit of a surprise to see where we're sleeping.

'Will this do?' May asks once we've practically folded our camp beds around the conference table. It's a very confined space.

'We'll manage,' Jonathan laughs as he unrolls the sleeping bags.

'You may have caught a whiff of it already,' May says, 'but next door is our spa area, where residents can swim.' When she sees my jaw drop in astonishment, she adds. 'That sounds fancier than it is. The previous owner of the house had it installed, and I thought: I bet our residents will appreciate that too, so we kept it in. Feel free to go for a dip if you like to chill for a bit, then we'll see you wandering out and about later, okay?'

The minute she's gone, Jonathan and I look at each other and say, in unison, 'this place isn't half bad.'

Once we've got ourselves settled in, we decide to save the pool for the evening and head upstairs. I go and sit with the residents, while Jonathan takes his camera outside to get some footage while the sun is out and bathes the house in beautiful light. I join a table where the florist is in the process of cutting fresh flowers.

'Aren't they gorgeous, all those colours?' I hear beside me. 'I'm Britta, and you?' My neighbour is talking to me in English, so she too must have figured that my curls aren't Danish.

'My name is Teun. And I'm glad you speak English, because it means we can have a nice chat,' I say with some relief, because I often worry about potential language barriers.

'Well, I prefer to speak German. My husband is from Germany, so it's almost a second language to me. Do you speak it?'

Because my first book is about to be published in all the German-speaking countries, I've just completed a German language course, but I wouldn't say I'm fluent yet. So I figure it would be good to get some practice in, and answer confidently: 'Of course I do. How do you like living here?'

She grabs hold of the armrests of her chair and sits up nice and straight. 'Life here is good, my boy. Obviously, most of the people are old and getting a bit shaky, but it's a nice place. Come, let me show you around and introduce you to the others.'

I don't need to be told twice. When I get to my feet, Britta gives me her hand and together we make our way outside. The first person we meet is Frederik, who's busy playing with the dog and barely even notices us. 'That's what usually happens when he bumps into his favourite pooch,' Britta says. 'We'll see him later at lunch.' Then we walk by the goats, who clearly know that where there are humans there might be a chance of food. The curious creatures come closer. 'Aren't they lovely?' Then it's on to the big hen house, where Torsten is generous with the feed and deep in conversation with the free-range chickens. 'Fresh eggs all year round,' I hear on my left, and I'm beginning to think that Britta isn't a resident, but a marketing manager. 'And here are the others, sitting round the fire pit. Hello everyone, this is Teun. He's come to stay here for a few days.' And with a deep sigh and a 'phew', she makes it clear that she considers her job done. 'Will you be alright?'

I shake her hand, which is still holding mine. 'Yes, absolutely, I've got this.'

Britta makes herself comfortable by the crackling fire that everybody has gathered round. I do the same and the woman next to me hands me a fleece blanket and says: 'For the raw sea wind.' I spend the rest of the afternoon chatting and getting to know the residents. Just about all of them strike me as lucid and alert. I'd love to know May's secret, I think as I close my eyes to enjoy the sun on my face, and before long the hubbub fades into the background.

In the days that follow I talk to the residents about their lives, eat restaurant-grade food, laugh at Britta, who grows jealous when the others chat to me for too long, listen to music by candlelight, and I see people sharing their bed with a cat they've brought from home, bobbing about in the pool and sinking into the massage chairs in the pristine white chill corner.

Just before we leave, I seek out May in the garden. 'So, what do you think? She's curious to know.

I need a moment to formulate my thoughts into words, because I'm still in two minds. 'First off, I have nothing but praise for this place you've created. Change requires courage, and I feel you have it in spades. I really admire that.' The compliment clearly means a lot to her. Next, I share my experience of the home. 'My overall feeling is one of wellness. It's like being pampered from morning till night.'

May looks pleased. 'That's our aim. We do all we can to give people a normal life.'

As we stroll around the garden, I ask about that one issue I'm so curious about: 'What strikes me is that almost everybody is lucid, that they laugh and cry and actively communicate with each other. How is that possible? What's the May Method?'

She's beaming with pride. 'I don't know if it's perfect care, because there are a lot of good places around the world, but it really works here.' Her blue eyes become even brighter. 'See, before I acquired this place, I'd always been struck by just how many people were staring apathetically into space or were sitting with their head slumped on the table. Whenever something happened, they'd react very briefly only to go vacant again. I tried to figure out why that was, and it became abundantly clear to me that the medication was to blame. Every time they were given medicine, they'd turn in on themselves, their eyes would glaze over, and it would be all but impossible to get through to them. That's what it is, I thought. So when I started my own place here, I began to reduce the doses, and I could see their eyes growing clearer, literally seeing the spark return.' What May has done is something that few people have the courage to do. But to my mind it's vital in the quest for a better quality of life, since apathy is such a big part of the current picture. 'These days we use hardly any medication and no sedatives at all, so we can communicate with almost everybody, even those who are non-verbal. It's so important to get rid of that glassy look and make eye contact. The eyes can tell you so much.' Sharp as she is, May concludes by asking: 'But what did you find less convincing, or what made you think 'hmm, why are they doing it like that?'

I decide to level with her and be just as honest about the negatives I experienced. 'What I noticed, and what I'm not sure about, is that people are waited on hand and foot all day. The staff deliberately adopt a subservient role, and that to me that completely overshoots the mark and makes the place feel more like a luxury boutique hotel than a real home.'

May listens attentively and waits for me to finish.

'It's something I can really enjoy, but after a week it would start to get on my nerves a bit. At home, if I were to snap my fingers every time I wanted a coffee or something to eat, I'd know what the response would be. And if no one ever says, "Why don't you do it yourself?" I'd probably turn into an obnoxious character and spoil the atmosphere. An unequal balance of power between people doesn't feel like a sustainable solution to me. Does that make sense?'

A look of doubt crosses her face, and then she says: 'The difficult thing is that I can't claim to know what people with dementia feel. But I do see when they're happy, so that's what I'm trying to aim for here. And whether that's ideal, I don't know, but so far it does feel like the best approach.'

I give her a cuddle and say: 'Thank you. I couldn't have expressed it better than that. It's remarkable to see that you put the residents' happiness at the heart of everything you do and give it your all. Keep doing what you do and keep searching and I'll do the same.'

We hug May one last time, say goodbye to everyone, pack up the camera, close the boot of the Volvo and drive back to the Netherlands with more clarity than we had on arrival.

VI Our hope

The paradox of growing awareness around dementia

South Africa

'Passports, please.' Jonathan and I hand our documents to the official in the immigration booth. 'Where are you going?' asks the young officer, who has to look up and down three times to see if the curly-headed guy in my passport is the same as the one he's facing right now.

'We're going to South Africa for a few weeks, and yes, that really is me in the photo.'

The stern look disappears. 'All right then, enjoy your visit. Next!'

I've been looking forward to this trip for ages. It feels like a real voyage of discovery. After months of phone calls, emails and WhatsApp messages during our preliminary research for the documentary, we established contact with researchers from around the world. But one of the biggest regions was never cited as an example of good care: Africa. It only made us more eager to explore this 'forgotten continent'. We discovered that this lack of attention is really rather peculiar, because United Nations data shows that in the years to come the elderly population in Africa is set to increase faster than in any other continent, which means that the number of people with some form of dementia is set to rise sharply too. This fact made us so curious about the way people in Africa approach dementia that we pulled out all the stops to try and add South Africa to our itinerary.

Through a series of Zoom calls we developed a good bond with a bunch of enthusiastic South African experts in the field of geriatrics (the specialism that deals with research into and treatment of the elderly with complex needs): Professor Jaco Hoffman (University of Oxford and North-West University in South Africa), Dr Adele van Wyk (University of the West of England) and Dr Rayne Stroebel (the founder of GERATEC), who've all done research into dementia in Africa as a whole and South Africa in particular. They mentioned the positive developments on the continent, but also the lack of awareness and the troubled cultural perception of dementia. In South Africa, only a small percentage of people with the condition end up in a nursing home, they told us, while the majority remain within the country's close-knit communities. The three scholars advised us to visit the townships to learn more about the culture and the reasons why things have panned out this way.

'You're kidding, Teun,' Jonathan says as I turn my hand luggage inside-out to find my passport for boarding.

'Did I not take it out of the tray at security?' I wonder in a bit of a panic.

'It's sticking out of your breast pocket, silly... Try not to lose something important while we're on the road, because Africa really is a different world.' He throws me an uncharacteristically serious look. Jonathan lived in South Africa for a few years, so I know he's not joking. 'If you apply common sense, you should be fine. You know, lots of Dutch people think it's strange that in South Africa you need to watch what you do, where you go and what you carry with you. But that changes as soon as you see for yourself what life there is like, and it dawns on you that our safe bubble in the Netherlands is the exception rather than the rule in the world at large.'

A little over twelve hours later, we're in a taxi in the dead of night, driving along the N2 from the airport to the centre of Cape Town. Thousands of little lights are suspended from the tangle of electricity cables on either side of the motorway, and underneath them are the faint contours of small huts. When the motorway starts twisting and turning and the lights make way for proper street lighting that reveals tree lined avenues and white townhouses, a voice from the front of the car tells us: 'We're nearly there.'

Jonathan leans forward and looks through the windscreen. 'In terms of landscape, this city has it all. Beautiful mountains, lots of greenery and right by the sea.'

We turn a corner and see the centre of Cape Town illuminated in the distance, giving us not only a sense of how big the city is, but also how Table Mountain provides a gorgeous backdrop for it.

The next morning I wake up early. I get out of bed and decide to go for a walk along the boulevard outside our hotel. Nearby, the waves crash furiously against big rocks in the ocean. It doesn't take me long to get a sense of the division in this country. I see the white population jogging in fancy attire and treating themselves to granola bowls and flat whites in trendy coffee bars, while black people pick up litter in the streets and whizz by in pickup trucks, about a dozen crammed into a cargo bed. If the differences are so huge at the best of times, then what's it like for vulnerable groups that need care, such as people with dementia?

When I arrive back at the hotel, looking like a drowned rat thanks to the sea spray, Jonathan is waiting in our car. He throws open the door. 'Look at the state of you. Get in quick. We've got a long journey ahead of us, so we'll stop for breakfast along the way, okay?'

I nod, sit down and lean back.

As we drive the city awakens, and on either side of the motorway I see what remained largely invisible in the dark last night: the townships. Names appear on the road signs – NYANGA, MITCHELL'S PLAIN and KHAYELITSHA – but to me it all looks like an endless plain with makeshift huts and houses constructed of a mishmash of materials. Plumes of smoke billow up into the sky, and through the open car window I catch the smell of burning rubbish.

En route we pass small Victorian villages with squeaky clean streets, beautiful, sprawling vineyards and palatial farms. Every now and then, this idyllic picture is rudely interrupted by yet another township. Nearly every town and village in South Africa has one or more, and they originate in the darkest period in the country's history: apartheid. We see a succession of extremes flashing past; rich and poor grow up against the same mountain backdrop here.

Some six hours later we take the exit for Thembalethu, the biggest township in the city of George. Most of the people in this 'black township' are Xhosas, one of the country's indigenous populations, known for their elegant click language. Our contact, Aunt Gloria, is highly respected in the community. When we reach a flyover, we suddenly find ourselves surrounded by a swarm of people and cars and scan the area for Tommy, a good friend of Aunt Gloria's, who will look after us during our stay.

Before long, lots of people gawp at the car with the two gesticulating white holiday-goers inside. Guys, most of them young, are jostling for position in the hope of being selected by older men holding up bits of paper. Work is so scarce here that getting hired for a day of physical labour is like winning the lottery. The 'lucky' ones jump in the back of small pickups and disappear down the motorway, before returning late at night with some pocket money. It's no surprise then that the crowd is astonished to see two unfamiliar faces in search of a place to park their car amidst the mayhem.

When Tommy turns up, he immediately twigs that we've become an attraction. He gestures nervously for us to remain seated, gets in the car and greets us with the words: 'Come, this is not the best place to hang around. We're heading that way.'

Once we've escaped the commotion, we get a good view of the township from the flyover and see that there's only one access road. I ask Tommy about it and he explains: 'Thembalethu has different zones, but you're right, there's only one entrance. It was designed that way, so the township could be hermetically sealed in case of trouble, which was done a lot by the apartheid commandos. These days, residents block the road, so the police can't get in.' A mischievous smile crosses his face. 'It's what I call karma.'

A few blocks on, we arrive in a small square with five houses. Guard dogs bark behind metal fences as we get out of the car. 'Don't worry, they're harmless,' Tommy reassures us, and together we enter Aunt Gloria's house. Two boys of about eight welcome us and take us by the hand and into the living room. From the kitchen we hear Aunt Gloria shout: 'Guys, is that you? I won't be a minute.'

In the living room a man sits on a large leather corner sofa. He rolls his eyes when we greet him. 'This is Joseph, Aunt Gloria's husband,' Tommy says. 'He suffered a stroke and since then he's had trouble remembering things.' When I try to have a chat with him, he just babbles and his absent gaze drifts to the TV – behaviour I often see at my nursing home and that strongly reminds me of a form of dementia.

'There you are, my boys from Holland. How wonderful to see you.' Aunt Gloria comes over to us in a gorgeous, colourful robe accessorised with a necklace of blue wooden beads. She's also wearing a tall fur hat and lightly tinted glasses, so I can't really see her eyes. Just as we're about to hug, she spots what we've brought along. 'Is that your video camera?' she asks, horrified.

'Er, yes? Is that a problem?' Jonathan asks.

'Umm, it could well become an issue. I thought you'd turn up with a small camera, not this enormous contraption. It will stand out, and you want to avoid that round here...'

During our drive over, Jonathan had already been fretting over the equipment. When he lived here, he never felt unsafe, not even in the townships, but back then he wasn't toting a very expensive video camera. 'It's like walking down the street with a bag of gold, trusting that nobody will notice. Fat chance! What we're about to do feels like Russian roulette...' We'd hoped to be safe with our contacts because we're here for a good cause, maar now that we're being told this on day one, I wonder what to expect in the coming weeks.

After a few phone calls with community leaders, we agree that we'll only head out in the company of Aunt Gloria. She's a respected figure and personally knows many of 'the killers', as she calls them. 'I used to be a teacher and taught most of those boys at one point or another. They won't hurt me, so hopefully you'll be alright too.'

I glance at Jonathan and I can tell he's thinking the same as me: hopefully... okay.

Luckily, Tommy, our designated driver and second chaperone, appears to be a lot more relaxed. 'It's gonna be fine, guys,' he says. 'I'm phoning the priest tomorrow to ask him what he thinks. For now, enjoy a cuppa, drop your luggage off at the hotel and have a good night's sleep.'

It feels bizarre to suddenly swap your sense of safety for fear and insecurity, and all that before the 'real work' has even begun. Jonathan and I raise our mugs to our lips, shrug our shoulders and lose ourselves in the cricket match on television. A few hours later, we say goodbye to Aunt Gloria and her family. It's pitch-black when we drop Tommy off at home and drive to our hotel, which is on the 'right and secure side' of the flyover.

That evening, Jonathan and I meet in the hotel bar for a drink and a debrief. The barman overhears us and adds some fuel to the flames: 'What? You're planning to film in Thembalethu?' He just about dies laughing. 'Whose idea was that? This is not the kind of touristy township you see on a tour in Cape Town or Johannesburg, you know? Thembalethu is the real deal, with very real people, who can be really dangerous.' He picks up a bottle or red wine and pours two glasses. 'I've lived there most of my life and let me tell you: it's not getting any better. The gangs that operate in there control everything. When it's your home, you learn to live with it, because that's just the way it is. But you whiteys?'

We allow ourselves to be carried away by his infectious laughter, even though we know that this is no laughing matter. When we tell him that until a few hours ago we were planning on sleeping in the township but found this place at the eleventh hour when we were advised not to, he slaps the bar, cracking up.

'What? You planned to spend the night there? Guys! In Thembalethu? Oh my God, I'm going to remember this till my dying day. Surely not in the hostel?'

We're feeling even more foolish now and nod sheepishly.

'Whatever next! They'd have left the back door wide open for all the "bad boys", and you'd have been dead by now. I'm sorry, guys, I don't mean to scare you. I'm sure you're in good hands with Aunt Gloria, but please be careful. I'm serious. The gang members show no mercy whatsoever and operate a strict "zero whites policy" these days. And they finish off everybody they rob or rape, so nobody can testify against them.'

I take a big sip of my wine and try to lighten the mood with a joke. 'Why don't you top up our glasses. They could well be our last.'

We raise another toast and laugh away our fears. Not much later, somewhat befuddled, we fall asleep.

The following morning we get into the car to collect Tommy and Aunt Gloria. We're tense. We'll be visiting some people who should be able to tell us more about the approach to cognitive problems in South African townships, as the term 'dementia' is all but unknown round here.

Aunt Gloria and Tommy crossed our path fairly early on during our preliminary enquiries into South Africa. They were introduced to us via Dr Adele van Wyk, who did research for her PhD in the region and received a great deal of help from them. Aunt Gloria collected her proverbial free bus pass a long time ago and is not so much an expert in care for the elderly, but in care generally. As someone who holds a prominent position in the Xhosa community, she knows exactly what's happening in the township, and also – more importantly – what's bubbling under the surface and who needs help the most. She works day and night, for as many different causes as she can manage. Whether it's food programmes, uniforms for school children or care for the elderly in the community, Aunt Gloria is always ready to help. As she told me during one of our preparatory Skype chats, 'I'm not rich by any means, but sharing is something I can do and love. It allows me to improve other people's lives, as well as my own'.

Our first stop is Norman, who lives behind Aunt Gloria and whose wife died just a week ago. He's waiting by the gate of his white stone house, chatting to his neighbour, while Tommy parks the car nearby. As soon as I approach, he goes inside and comes back with a framed photo of his wife. 'She was the most beautiful woman in the world,' he says. 'She was everything to me, but now she's gone. God has taken her because her time had come.' A tear rolls down his face as he gazes at the picture.

I see that he needs this moment of silence and look intently at the image. After about a minute, I say: 'She looks beautiful, and strong too.'

The corners of Norman's mouth turn upwards ever so slightly. 'Yes, she certainly was! A lioness. It's why she was mayor of Thembalethu for a long time. It may not be a title that's officially recognised outside the township walls, but in here it's the highest possible honour.'

With the loss still so fresh, I ask tentatively: 'Had your wife been ill for a long time?'

He sighs, and I see despair in his eyes. 'It's so strange. She passed away, but nobody seems to know exactly what the cause was. Her head wasn't right, the doctor said, but there was nothing they could do.' He heaves another sigh. 'She was given so many different medications, but none of them helped. She became more and more forgetful, woke up frightened during the night and didn't want to leave the house anymore, because she couldn't understand what was happening to her.' Norman shakes his head. 'My once mighty lioness, who wasn't afraid of anything or anyone, turned into a fearful little kitten. It just doesn't make sense to me. So maybe it's for the best. Now she finally gets to enjoy her well-earned rest.' He looks at me with sorrow in his eyes and now all he can do is nod. I feel it's becoming too hard for him to talk.

I nod back, say goodbye with a big hug and tell him: 'What an amazing wife you had. Thank you for telling me about her.'

A faint smile appears on his face, and when we leave I see that he's still standing by the gate, clutching his wife's photo under his arm – an image I won't forget in a hurry.

I've ended up in a world that's different in every respect: not just in terms of affluence, facilities and safety, but also when it comes to health care. I feel that in the Netherlands we'd keep searching until there's a diagnosis. When confronted with symptoms, I'd expect to find a cause and wouldn't settle for 'your head's not right'. At the same time, I wonder if Norman and his wife would have been happier had they known that she was probably suffering from a form of dementia. It's not an easy question to answer, because in our country the label dementia all too often leads to isolation, shame, exclusion, confinement and ultimately even social death.

For our next stop, we turn off the bigger paved road and park the car on a patch of grass with three dilapidated buildings and a few small children playing with a broken wheelbarrow.

As soon as I get out and hear the women's choir, I get goosebumps. Through the small windows of the low chalk-coloured structure, I see them dancing and clapping to lively, uplifting music. Luckily that doesn't change when we enter, and a man standing in front of the choir encourages me to join in. It's as if the music welcomes me with open arms and instantly includes me in the group. The harmonies carry me, and the energy of the forty elderly women pushes everything else to the background. I'm no longer afraid of external dangers, but feel happy and privileged to be here.

Half of the large room is filled with about fifty plastic chairs, while the rest is used for ball games and other exercises, which are also accompanied by song. In the breaks between the singing and dancing, soup is served from the adjacent kitchen, and I talk to the ladies in the chairs about old age. Like my housemates, they tell me that everything is happening faster and faster, but aside from that they're really happy with the life that's been granted them. Not least because of this meeting place, where they like to gather to talk about serious and less serious matters. Mention of the latter, especially, elicits loud whooping and hollering.

'Yes, young man, we talk about absolutely everything round here!' yells the most gregarious one, while the other women leave no doubt as to what topic she's referring to by giggling even more.

I smile and play along: 'What do you make of the guy in the cap?'

The ladies whoop louder.

When we're done clowning around and I enquire if they know anyone who suffers from forgetfulness, nearly all hands go up. And when asked if that ever leads to awkward situations, most hands stay up.

'Why do you want to know?' a woman in the front row asks.

'Good question!' I say. 'I'm trying to find out what other countries can teach us about the subject of dementia. Do you know what that is?'

No hands go up this time.

'Nobody? There are lots of different forms of dementia, but the best-known one is Alzheimer's. The people who have it, who are mostly older, start to forget things, which gets worse over time.'

I see many of them nodding in recognition and conferring with their neighbours.

'I'd love to hear what you think about it and what we can do to give people the best possible future.'

The most gregarious one walks up to the front and says: 'It's good to hear that you want to talk about this. I think many of us recognise it either in ourselves or in someone close to us, so please all of you come forward and talk to this young man. He's travelled all the way from the Netherlands for this.'

In the hours that follow, everybody shares their story. For many women, it seems to be a revelation or a relief to know that they're not alone. I hear about a man who often visits the local store and when he can't find his way back is taken home by another customer or the shopkeeper himself without anyone complaining or wondering what's going on. I also hear about an elderly woman who's always talking to herself when she walks around the neighbourhood, and about a man who claims to see things that are invisible to others. But I hear no judgement in any of their voices. They've noticed the behaviour, but it never occurred to them that it might be something specific.

'It's just part of life. Everybody is different, right? Old age comes with frailty, we all know and feel that,' a woman says, and everybody loudly concurs. 'Round here we take life one day at a time. That's something we've learned to do, and it feels right. Be grateful for the time you're given, because it's over before you know it.'

Whereupon they all rise to their feet and start clapping and cheering.

As I'm saying goodbye to each of the forty ladies, one woman introduces herself as Rose, and she invites me over to her house for a chat. I leap at the opportunity. Rose is wearing a gorgeous headscarf and a vintage Champion hoodie, which has seen better days. She explains that she's walked a long way, and we decide to follow her on foot, with Tommy and Aunt Gloria making up the rear in the car, for protection.

Five minutes later, Rose is walking ahead of me, with Jonathan filming her. Gradually, more and more young men start trailing us, until Tommy shouts: 'Get in, now!' Rose remains calm and keeps going, but I don't take any chances and jump in the car. Jonathan quickly makes his way over as well. Two cars approach. From the back seat of our car, Aunt Gloria yells: 'Watch out, guys, it's them! The killers!' Pale as a sheet, Jonathan manages to get in just before we're cut off by the two brightly coloured cars that look like they've been through the wars. Two big guys with tattooed faces get out of a purple Toyota Corolla with a cracked windscreen and dented side panels in a variety of shades.

'Keep calm, I'll do the talking,' Aunt Gloria says.

The men peer in through the open windows, and the biggest turns to Jonathan, who's in the back. 'Hey, how's it going? Nice thing you've got there.'

Jonathan refuses to be intimidated and says in a friendly tone of voice: 'I know, right? I really like it too.'

Aunt Gloria intervenes and yells something short and sharp in Xhosa at the man, who looks up and immediately turns his attention to her. He clearly recognises Aunt Gloria. She wastes no time and addresses the men like a tough and cold-blooded mafia boss. Without moving anything other than her mouth, she calmly tells the men in English that they've got no business here, and that she'll enlist everybody she knows to teach them a lesson if they think otherwise. 'And you know who I mean, right?' she says menacingly.

The man at the car window laughs like a hyena, a high-pitched cackle that reveals the golden grill on his teeth. 'Okay, okay, Aunt. You know we'd never hurt anyone.' When both men smile at us, I feel cold shivers down my spine. 'We're just keeping an eye on you, no more, no less, all right?' Their final glance tells us that they're dead serious, and then they're back in their car and off.

'If it wasn't for me, you'd be dead by now,' Aunt Gloria notes calmly and then casually asks Tommy: 'Shall we?'

I lean back in the passenger seat and in the side-view mirror I see Jonathan sitting wanly in the back. He appears to be in shock. 'You okay, Jonathan? That was a close call, wasn't it?'

'Holy shit, man! I've seen a lot in my life, but I've never been this close to death before.' He turns to the hero of the day. 'You're a real boss, Aunt Gloria. Thank you for the rescue operation.'

Gloria shrugs her shoulders and says what people in Africa often say when something weird or wonderful happens: 'TIA. This is Africa.'

We all laugh.

We drive deeper into the neighbourhood until we arrive at a terracotta-coloured bungalow, where Rose is waiting for us. The first thing we notice when she opens the front door are the bits of tarpaulin that cover the bare ground. Rose walks over to a glass display case and shows us photos of her children, which have been arranged in front of a kind of mini altar. She has outlived them: her eldest daughter was found murdered, while her youngest died of an overdose. Now that she's all alone, everyday life is much harder, not least because she's becoming more and more forgetful. That's what she wants to talk to me about. The questions she puts to me are suffused with the hope that I have a solution.

'Dear Rose, this isn't something I can solve for you,' I say in a bid to manage her expectations. 'But what kind of help are you getting here? What are they telling you?'

With a deep sigh, she starts talking. 'Doctor Brewe at the hospital says it's because I think too much. "No, lady, you think too much. What's going on with you, tell us."' She has a desperate look in her eyes. 'Sometimes I don't know what's going on, I really don't,' she continues, and plonks down in her large armchair. 'I'm old and lead a simple life. I don't have much to lose, because I've already lost what I held dearest. So I hope I can make the most of the time I have left. That's why I'm so pleased with my nephews, who come and bring me water or a bowl of rice from time to time, a chat with the neighbours, the cows from up the road that I see every once in a while, my friends at the women's club, who are always up for a laugh. It's a small life, but it's big and good enough for me. I hope my head won't forget that.'

Since my arrival in this country, I've been on a rollercoaster of emotions, which reached its climax in this township. Intense happiness and sorrow have taken dizzying turns. Despite the situation they're in, people here seem to have this indestructible hope and even see dementia as a minor problem so long as they can still enjoy the little things in life.

I realise that in the Netherlands we often lose sight of these small joys during the final stages of life, what with all our care, innovation and technology. But when you listen carefully, those are not the things that people are after when they ask for help. Professor Anne-Mei The puts it very well: 'People ask for the best possible life, but the answer we give them is care. Care is good for a lot of things, but it doesn't always lead to happiness, and that's something we need to bear in mind when people say: help me. We must learn to listen to the actual need instead of trying to fill it with care.'

When twilight starts to fall, Aunt Gloria says it's time to go. I get to my feet and give Rose three kisses, a cuddle and a bit of money for rice. 'You're an inspiration to me, Rose. I hope that one day I'll be just as grateful as you.'

She wraps her arms around my waist, presses her head against me and says: 'Thank you for coming to us. Africa won't forget you.'

I get into the car with tears in my eyes, not sure if I'm crying for joy or sorrow. This really is the most bizarre day ever, I think to myself, as the setting sun paints the corrugated metal roofs blood red and Aunt Gloria dozes off in the back seat.

A few days later we're joined by social workers and Pastor Akhona who, like Aunt Gloria, is a highly respected figure in the community. Our car hasn't become any bigger though, so as we drive through the township, the seven of us are very 'snug' in our four-seater.

After fifteen minutes, Tommy stops, and the pastor exclaims: 'Welcome to Silvertown!' We get out and follow him into a large slum. He explains: 'This part of the township gets its name from all the corrugated metal huts that make this side of the hill shimmer like silver in the afternoon sun.' Huts is the right word. Barely three by three metres, they're formed of three iron sheets that are riveted together, topped with a fourth that serves as the roof. There's rubbish everywhere. Small fires burn beside laundry that's hung up to dry between the huts, and chickens and their young wander into the road in search of food. People go about barefoot, in broken shoes or a combination of the two, and look wary when our group passes.

'This is one of those places where God really tests your faith,' the pastor says, looking sad. We're standing beside a field dotted with crosses. 'The people who live here fight death on a daily basis and are often defeated. There's no food around here, no drinking water, no services, nothing, except a few silver-coloured sheets that, if you're lucky, you can call home.

We're silent as we look at the makeshift graveyard and the shockingly recent birth years on the crosses.

'Come, we'll let them rest in peace,' the pastor says.

We walk on through smelly alleyways, where emaciated cats and dogs roam about and small children peer curiously through cracks between the walls.

'We know an elderly woman down here who's becoming increasingly forgetful and is struggling to look after herself,' one of the social workers tells us.

On top of the hill we take a left turn down a narrow passageway between two houses, where we have to walk bent over so we don't knock our heads against any loose corrugated sheeting or other construction materials. When we reach the end, we squeeze past two wooden planks that look like they're meant to conceal the entrance to the alley and find ourselves on a patch of grass with four ramshackle huts.

A woman sits on the ground in front of the most dilapidated one. She looks up in a daze when she becomes aware of us and then stares down again. I squat and see that white crusts have formed in the corners of her mouth due to dehydration.

I grab my bottle. 'Please, have some water. You need to drink.'

The woman looks at me as if to say: really? She's so weak she can barely unscrew the cap, so I do it for her. Her hands tremble as she raises the bottle to her lips and much of the water gushes down her chin. But she heaves a deep sigh when she manages to swallow a little. Slowly, very slowly, she perks up a bit and mumbles: 'Thank you.' We remain seated a while so she can get her strength back up and then we help her inside, out of the sun. There's a bed in the middle of the hut and an old stereo and chamber pot next to it. Together they all but take up the entire space.

After the social worker gives her a cracker, she tells us that she hasn't had anything to eat for eight days, her vision was blurred and she had to sit down when she felt dizzy outside.

'Eight days without food?' I say out loud, and it dawns on me that this here is life in its most elemental form. I don't know what to say to the woman, because absolutely everything feels inappropriate.

When I sit down next to her on the bed and take her rough hands in mine, she suddenly starts talking: 'Normally I collect plastic caps at the rubbish dump. That earns me seven cents a week. That's usually just enough for a bit of water or a small sandwich bag of rice, but these days I often feel unwell, so that means I can't earn any money and don't have any food.'

Again, I don't know what to say to someone who only moments ago was practically dying of hunger and thirst and is now grateful for a bit of water. I feel ashamed on behalf of all those in the Netherlands who have the audacity to dismiss you as an 'economic migrant' when you flee this kind of situation. You're not a fortune seeker when staying where you are equals death. It pains me that we just can't seem to get our heads round the fact that we aren't more entitled to the best possible life than people who were born elsewhere.

It's as if we're simply not prepared to share. We were born here, in safety and prosperity, so we deserve all this. But what do people who were born in war and poverty deserve? The sheer hopelessness I sense in this township is truly indescribable. How can I look this woman in the eye and explain that we, with everything we have, can't do any more for her than we already do? Is it any surprise that folks in such circumstances want to escape to a place where people seem to have it all?

Even though we agreed not to take any more unnecessary risks after our first experience of intimidation, in the afternoon our social worker friends persuade us to visit the dangerous heart of Thembalethu, Zone 6. They've noticed that word of our presence has spread via the jungle drums in recent days, and many people are curious. Among them is a woman who has been looking after her mother with 'special symptoms' for many years. She'd love to talk to me about it, and of course I don't want to pass up the opportunity and honour. We pluck up all our courage, get into the cramped car and enter the notorious zone.

It's immediately clear that living conditions in this part of the township are equally wretched. Everywhere we look, we see rundown old cars from bygone eras and barbed wire fencing off patches of land on which small, caved-in houses accommodate entire families. With each gust of cool air, red sand blows through the streets. A group of children run ahead of the car and seem to know exactly where we're going. When we get out just up the road, our team immediately implements some precautionary measures. While Jonathan and I make our way to the house, Tommy and the social workers position themselves at either end of the street, and one person stays in the car with Aunt Gloria, so we can drive away at short notice. It's bizarre how quickly this has come to feel normal, I think to myself, as we're welcomed behind the tall chicken-wire fence. Daughter Khetiwe, wearing a brightly-coloured apron, stands in front of the turquoise hut that is just about held together with wooden planks. She gives us a warm hug. Sitting next to her on a stack of car tyres, in a blue wool winter coat, is her mother Qaqamba.

Khetiwe is so keen to share her story that she launches straight in. She tells us that at first her mother would forget the odd thing, but now has little or no awareness of anything she says or does.

'How do you feel about your mother's memory loss?' I ask in English.

She glances up at the sky as she searches for the right words. 'I'm not sure, but I think it's part of old age. I don't know what it's like to be elderly, but I see lots of others struggle with the same thing and, like my mother, talk to themselves.' Khetiwe slides closer to her mother to give her a cuddle, and then continues: 'When I'm working outside or lying in bed, I'll hear her say all kinds of things and I'll ask: "Mum, what is it? Who are you talking to?" But then as soon as I go to her, she'll look at me all innocently and won't know what

I mean. She never used to do that, but it's getting worse now at her advanced age.' Again, she looks lovingly at her mother, but when she turns to face me her tone suddenly changes. 'I often tell my mother: "You better be careful with all this talking to yourself, because this is why young guys are killing old people. They'll think you're a witch."'

That last sentence comes out so casually that it takes about ten seconds to sink in.

'A witch?' I ask.

Khetiwe's serious demeanour doesn't change. 'Yes, many people in these parts still believe in witchcraft. That's why I'm so scared they'll murder my mother. A woman I knew in the next village was murdered because she was suspected of being a witch. They set her house alight with her still in it and when she ran out they kicked and beat her back in so she'd burn alive. And that's exactly what happened. It burnt down to the ground, with her inside.' Khetiwe rubs her teary eyes. 'That's why you must have a good caretaker, someone who takes good care of my mum and watches over her.'

'So the decision to look after your mother is really a matter of life and death?' I ask.

She starts crying and nods.

Shaken, I stand up to comfort her. 'Hang in there, dear Khetiwe. You're a strong woman.' She drops her shoulders and for a moment she's limp in my arms.

I'm trying to process what I've just heard. It's the total opposite of the other experiences I've had in this country. Nowhere else in the world have I seen people, at whatever stage of dementia, remain part of their community. In many cases 'challenging' behaviour is accepted; it may be puzzling, but because these people belong to a close-knit group it stands to reason that they're looked after. While the lack of a label doesn't seem to make their lives any easier, it does create some space in their twilight years for a bit of happiness, and it's up to them to decide what that looks like. It has helped me see that 'not knowing' isn't necessarily a negative thing, but it's a different story when not knowing means you may be tarred with a label that could put your life in danger, as in Khetiwe's mother's case. When that happens it's actually really important that people learn about dementia. This paradox of growing awareness is something I've never really thought about before.

Perhaps the solution lies not so much in raising awareness of dementia as in debunking dangerous myths, such as a belief in witchcraft. Instead of swapping one label for another, the majority who thankfully don't believe in witches can try to convince those that do that the misunderstood behaviour they're seeing isn't supernatural but only too human. If we do that, without linking it to prejudices, labels or fears, I'm sure people will be treated more humanely.

A label is by definition dangerous, all the more so in a society that aspires to perfection, in which physical beauty, financial success and academic excellence are seen as the ultimate goals, and that certainly seems to be the case in our country. Because one thing is certain: if you deviate from the norm and acquire a label, you can be assured of a life full of negative consequences, ranging from minor to life-threateningly big, like here.

After we've said goodbye to Khetiwe and her mother and we drive off again, Aunt Gloria sees our upset faces. 'Dear boys,' she says, 'now you've seen for yourselves that life here is very hard. But you've also noticed that most people still experience a lot of happiness. And do you know why? Because of Thembalethu, which means "our hope".' Her eyes beam with pride. 'We believe that today is a gift and tomorrow will be better, so whatever happened in the past and however hard things are right now, they'll never take our hope from us.'

VII Algorithms and superfood

The quiet revolution that is prevention

Sweden – South Korea

Because I don't want my contact with Ad to fizzle out, I still swing by regularly so we can pop out for a coffee or a beer. On the last two occasions I noticed that he'd become a little morose again. When I asked him about it, he replied: 'The old gang is getting worse. Elly is gone, Tineke can barely speak, and I hear that Murielle isn't doing so well in her new home. Wouldn't it be nice if you could give them a pill and cure them all?'

'Absolutely, Ad, I can see why you'd think that,' I said, while a gloomy Ad took a sip of his beer at our old local, Ouwe Dikke Dries.

As part of my search for ways to improve the quality of life for dementia sufferers, I speak to lots of scientists, but so far I haven't really considered the biomedical side of things. That's partly because 'finding the cure' has been the world's main focus for decades, but even more so because to date this has had little or no impact on the happiness of people who currently live with a form of dementia. And that happiness is exactly why I wanted to broaden my horizon and look at the international picture. So during our preliminary research I'm surprised to find myself gripped by the phenomenon of prevention. But while it's part of the biomedical field, it doesn't seek to cure dementia; it just looks at ways to prevent future cases of the disease.

I've never actually seen for myself how much some countries and organisations have done in the area of prevention, but after a chat with Professor Gill Livingston from the UK I'm keen to learn more. A while ago, she told me that prevention doesn't receive the attention it deserves, even though some methods of preventing or reducing the risk of dementia are extremely effective. To my amazement, those methods can even be used to slow the decline of cognitive function post-diagnosis. The facts and contacts she shared with us gave our research a new angle and moved it up a gear.

A few months later I'm in contact with researchers from around the globe who are part of FINGERS. This worldwide network for risk reduction and prevention of dementia brings together research teams from over forty countries and is led by a Finnish neuroscientist, Professor Miia Kivipelto. She's the network's founder and set up the ground-breaking FINGER study, the Finnish Geriatric Intervention Study to Prevent Cognitive Impairment and Disability. It has identified five areas that together form the basis for a preventative approach to dementia, like five fingers forming a hand: healthy food, physical exercise, mental stimulation, social activities and monitoring of vascular risk. Intervention in these lifestyle factors can delay cognitive decline and even improve performance in specific cognitive domains in people at risk of developing dementia. The FINGER method has become the worldwide blueprint for risk reduction and prevention.

It's obvious that I have to go and see Miia.

Since the coronavirus pandemic shows no sign of easing, it's a huge challenge, but eventually we manage to travel to the renowned Karolinska Institute in Stockholm. The hospital corridors stop feeling cold as soon as Miia, a vivacious and stylish woman in her forties, greets us enthusiastically. Bonding over our shared love of people with dementia, we get into a great conversation. She's particularly interested in my remarkable domestic set-up. 'One of the things I always say at the start of a lecture is that you're never too young to change, so what you're doing is perfect! In our society, we get out of the habit of exploring, discovering and learning new things. From the age of around forty you start preparing for retirement. You reduce your hours, maybe do less challenging jobs and go down the path of "dozing off", as I call it. If there's one thing that's bad for our brains it's that. So remember, even if you stop working, make sure your head doesn't! Keep making new connections in your brain, because that's what keeps it young.' She pauses, sips some water and then resumes: 'And the great thing is: it's free, so everyone can do it. We just need to make sure that we reach people all over the world.'

'That sounds very promising,' I reply. 'But is it really that simple?'

'Yes, it's that simple. Right now, we're seeing that 40 percent of all cases of dementia are linked to lifestyle factors that are within our control to change, and that means that some of those cases could be prevented. And given that we're currently looking at further risk factors for cognitive decline – such as depression, despair, loneliness, sleep disturbances, stress as well as air pollution – I suspect the percentage of cases that may be preventable will be even higher in the future.'

'That's incredible, but why do we hear so little about this?'

A smile spreads across her face. 'That's what I'd like to know. But luckily change is imminent, as more and more major players, such as the World Health Organization and a commission affiliated with the prestigious medical journal *The Lancet* [made up of a global team of leading experts from a range of disciplines] have embraced dementia prevention. So if we work together and put all five fingers into practice we should be able to manage the coming dementia epidemic much better.'

In the hours that follow, Miia talks passionately about her mission and I come away with a much clearer idea of what the method entails, how it works in practice and what it might mean for the future. Here's a brief summary of the five-pronged approach of the FINGER method:

1. *Physical exercise.* Think not just sport, but any kind of movement. It's very important to avoid sitting down too much and for too long at a time, and to get up and move around and incorporate some sort of activity into your day, such as walking, taking the stairs instead of the lift, going for a short bike ride, etc. It may not sound ground-breaking, but these brief moments of mobility are essential.

2. *Healthy food.* Our brain needs a lot of nutrients, so eating well is essential. If you can, eat foods that are part of the MIND diet, which combines the Mediterranean and low-salt DASH diets and contains plenty of green leafy vegetables, healthy fats from fish and olive oil, nuts, berries and beans. Drink lots of water and avoid fried foods, sugar, salt, red meat and dairy.

3. *Mental stimulation.* The brain is a muscle that needs exercise throughout life. So keep your mind active, learn new things and seek out fresh challenges. It's a simple case of use it or lose it. It's particularly important to stimulate your brain when you're getting older and you no longer work.

4. *Social activities, spending time with others, sleep management and stress management.* The pandemic showed that social activities are even more important for brain health than previously thought. Ask neighbours, family and friends to pop over every once in a while when you're old or in need of help. Avoid isolation and let the outside world in.

5. *Vascular risk monitoring.* A healthy vascular system is critical to the prevention of dementia, so make sure you do everything you can to avoid high blood pressure, diabetes and obesity. Here too a simple rule applies: what's good for your heart is good for your brain.

Tackling these risk factors is central to the FINGER method, which is good news because technically anyone anywhere in the world can start cutting their risk of developing dementia right now. But to boost the chances of this actually happening, we need to invest heavily in awareness campaigns around dementia prevention. This is particularly urgent in low and middle-income countries, which, according to the latest figures, are expected to see the fastest rise in people with dementia in the coming years.

A crucial component is the adaptation of the FINGER method for other cultural settings. There are huge differences worldwide in how and what we eat, how we exercise and socialise and how we learn new things. The FINGERS network now focuses on implementing new models to encourage their use around the world.

One country that has elevated local implementation to an art form, according to Miia, is South Korea, which has not only adopted the method, but has taken it a step further. 'We were wondering just now why we hear so little about dementia prevention, but in Korea that hasn't been the case for some time now. It's the only country in the world that has made it a national priority,' she tells me, beaming.

I can't help but think: we have to go there.

When we say goodbye and I thank her for the pleasant and invaluable conversation, she grabs me by the arm and says: 'Remember guys, what I said at the start is true. The road to dementia often begins some twenty to thirty years prior to diagnosis, so you're never too young to start changing. Please spread the word during your adventure.'

After our visit to Stockholm, we're really keen to see this 'new world' of prevention for ourselves, but the resurgent pandemic puts paid to our plans. A few months pass before we're given the green light by the South Korean government, and we quickly book a flight before the situation changes again. Our visit is, however, subject to one important condition: on arrival we have to spend a week in quarantine. It's not something we'd normally do on account of planning issues and costs, but after our many failed attempts to go to South Korea we take it in our stride, without giving too much thought to how it will all unfold on the other side of the world.

After a suspiciously empty flight, during which we have the enormous Boeing almost to ourselves, we land at Seoul airport. The first thing we notice is that the country operates an entirely different coronavirus policy. When we emerge from the airbridge, we see big colourful noticeboards everywhere featuring face masks and warning signs, so the place looks more like a disaster site than an airport. Soldiers in white 'spacesuits', complete with face coverings, wave their arms to direct everybody to the right desk. Nobody protests. You can tell people are used to obeying such orders, whereas for us this display of authority comes as a bit of a shock, to put it mildly.

As in Moldova, we're the only foreigners and here too we're plucked out of the queue and subjected to a thorough check. Then, with our official documentation stamped, we're taken to a specially designated 'corona hotel'. There we're met by more military personnel, again in white hazmat suits, a spectacle made all the more dramatic by big black machine guns. To inject a bit of levity into the pretty unusual check-in procedure, we try to fool around a bit, but that's clearly not appreciated. 'Silence!' comes the order from behind the desk.

Because we don't know what to expect in these turbulent times and we'll be crisscrossing the country, we've added Jonathan's business partner and our mutual friend, Bastiaan, to our team. Initially we're a bit embarrassed because these are his first impressions of our research, but a little later we can't stop laughing at the sight of him being turned inside-out in the supersonic 'car wash' of our 'cosy' quarantine hotel. 'Fun, isn't it, travelling with us?' Jonathan quips.

The flippancy is short-lived when we learn that we're all in separate rooms and that there's to be no contact between us whatsoever. We're alerted to the various security cameras in the corridor, which will keep an eye on us day and night. We're only allowed to open our room door when the buzzer sounds for our meals, which will be left outside in a white plastic bag three times a day. Finally, we're told to report our body temperature twice a day via an app, which we have to install right there and then. If you're late, you're out on your ear and on a flight home. And so, five minutes in, our picture of a week chilling together in a hotel is shattered. In shock, and clutching our first bag of food, we each enter our room, which now feels like a prison cell.

Never before have I felt the walls close in on me as I do in the days that follow, when we can only check in on each other by shouting through the cantilever windows. With little or no mobile reception, we're completely isolated in our nine square metres with a bed, shower and Korean TV. I hear you thinking that I should be used to being confined, but I've never experienced anything like it. Spending our days lying in bed and pacing our rooms is doing our heads in much sooner than we thought.

So this is what it feels like to be properly locked up, I think to myself. Just then I'm startled by the loud mealtime buzzer, and I hear us opening our doors one by one so as to avoid one another in the corridor. Needless to say, the first evening we all did it at the same time, upon which our phones pinged in unison, threatening us with deportation. We scurried back into our rooms and kept our heads down after that. It was the moment when any last bit of joy was sucked out of us, leaving nothing but a weird sense of doom.

Our highlight of the day comes when the internet briefly works and we share creative photos of the kimchi and white rice we're served three times a day (kimchi is a traditional Korean dish made of fermented cabbage and vegetables). I keep seeing parallels between my room here and the one in my nursing home. When you've got nothing to do all day, meals are the only moment to look forward to, but when the food is just as lacklustre as you are, I'm not surprised that my housemates end up literally sleeping face-down on their plates.

When we're 'released' a week later, to the minute, our muscles have trouble adjusting as we walk to the lift, so we all arrive at reception with wobbly sea legs. Wobbly after a week of sitting still? Now I can say more confidently what I've been saying all along: we're making people worse than they already are! If I've got trouble standing up after a week of immobility, it's really no surprise that most of my housemates, who are always sitting still, use a walking frame after a few weeks and not much later trundle around the house in a wheelchair. It's not exactly rocket science, so why can't the medical establishment come up with something better than to reduce people in the final stage of life to battery hens?

Do we all want to wither away when it's our turn? I think not. Then why is it so hard to enthuse our care sector for a more active final phase, when it adds so much to the happiness and quality of life of residents? My trip to Sweden has taught me that there's certainly no lack of evidence for its effectiveness. Let's see how they tackle it here.

After the person behind the desk hands me back my passport, I roll my suitcase outside and finally feel the wind in my hair again.

An hour's taxi ride later we reach Seoul, and the sun comes out, both literally and figuratively, the minute we enter this bustling city. I marvel at the street life and the smells that waft in through the open windows. It never ceases to amaze me just how quickly your mind and body adapt. A few hours earlier, we'd come out of our solitary confinement still totally dejected, but now the vibe in the car is like that on the first day of summer camp.

At the hotel, we check into a family room for the remainder of our stay, drop off our things and then quickly make our way to a surprise organised by one of our contacts. Strolling among the skyscrapers that rise up into the heavens on either side of the street, I'm infused with a renewed sense of adventure, even more so when Google Maps leads us to a basement restaurant.

The joint is thick with smoke and all those present look up as one when we enter. A man in the centre of the room jumps to his feet and shouts: 'Finally, there you are, guys! Come join us.' It's Solomon, our contact. All the tables are covered in glistening bowls and small barbecues, with diners grilling vegetables and thinly sliced meat.

When we reach our table, Solomon says: 'This is *soju*, a Korean rice wine that our ancestors used to drink at New Year to ward off disease and evil spirits, but today we're drinking it to forget about your first week here. The word *soju* means "welcoming spring", so welcome to Korea, my new friends!'

We clink glasses, and the barbecue on our table is fired up again for us.

Solomon Han is a successful businessman and looks the part too. He's like a Korean version of Apple founder Steve Jobs: black turtleneck, black trousers, shiny black shoes and stylish specs with thin frames. Having started several companies, in recent years he has turned his attention to collecting and processing medical data on dementia. Using artificial intelligence, he then converted this information into algorithms for the prevention and reduction of cognitive decline before combining the various algorithms into a 24-week programme with the evocative name SUPERBRAIN (SoUth

Korean study to PrEvent cognitive impaiRment and protect BRAIN health through lifestyle intervention in at-risk elderly people).

The day after a cathartic evening of socialising, we drop by the headquarters of Team Superbrain, which is located in the city centre on one of the upper floors of a gleaming glass skyscraper. Looking out over Seoul's central station, which is nearly a hundred years old and presents a beautiful contrast with the modern skyline, I talk to Solomon about his company. 'Superbrain is the world's first digital therapy to target multiple areas to prevent dementia,' he explains. 'The therapy was developed by leading South Korean scientists who spent decades doing research in this field. It's the combination of their knowledge, our programme and close collaboration with the government that has enabled us to get dementia prevention on people's radar – with the aim of improving or stabilising quality of life.'

I ask him: 'How is it possible that you've been working on this for so long, while we hear so little about it in the west?'

Solomon gives an understanding nod. 'It's certainly no coincidence that dementia is such a focal point in South Korea, because recent studies have shown that by 2044 we'll be the most aged country in the world. And with all the IT expertise we have here, we soon realised that the digital world might be able to provide a solution to a physical problem. Precisely because it's still not a priority in many countries, we're proud to be sharing our knowledge with you and the rest of the world. Hopefully it will top the agenda soon.'

His persuasive words are making me even more curious to know how this method of prevention works in practice, so I gladly accept a tour of the company. As he's showing me round, I keep thinking that I've ended up at Microsoft headquarters instead of at the birthplace of dementia prevention. We pass offices filled with clever computer programmers and software developers who are led by an enormous research and development department. I have to say, though, it does raise a whole bunch of new questions, because technological developments so often pan out differently in practice. Take the introduction of the illustrious Tovertafel, literally magic table, for example. Sold to aid social interaction, it can project digital creatures such as butterflies and fish for people to touch and follow. It was designed as a fun activity for people who sit a lot and to stimulate mobility. In practice, however, it stops people from getting up from their chairs or from going outside, and the butterflies and fish end up confusing them. It means that in most of the homes I've visited, the well-meaning contraption has become an expensive dust magnet.

In search of answers to my questions, we're going to have a look at the situation on the ground in South Korea and talk to the scientists at the forefront of this quiet digital revolution. Our next stop is a dementia centre, a grey and fairly average looking office building. At four storeys high, it feels small because of the surrounding towers. On the top floor we're met by three doctors in white coats, who bow in unison when we introduce ourselves.

Although you can get by with English in many places in Korea, the older generations are less familiar with the language. To overcome any linguistic barriers, Team Superbrain has arranged for an interpreter who often works for international film crews. Hannah, a vivacious and well-travelled young woman in her thirties, will be accompanying us wherever we go. She shows us what she's made of from the outset. Not only does she impress with her language skills, but she also introduces us to the rules of etiquette by demonstrating how to respond with the correct bow.

Following a brief introduction by the senior physicians, I'm handed a hi vis vest and find myself in an exercise class with people who are at least as old as my housemates, so I feel right at home.

When people in Korea turn sixty, they receive an official invitation to voluntarily register with one of the country's 220 dementia centres. With the help of several tests – including physical (how fit are you?), cognitive (how good and fast are your reasoning, information-processing, problem-solving, reaction, maths and reading skills?) and vascular (screening for blood sugar, hypertension, BMI, etc.) – they're then assessed for potential risk factors for developing dementia. Those who meet the criteria can immediately embark on the 24-week digital programme, which is aimed at making lifestyle changes using the five pillars of the FINGER method. The programme tracks progress in each area and helps participants, step by step, reach the next phase.

The dementia centre fulfils an essential role in the programme, as it's where many of the changes are explained and people can gather to practice together. I get to witness one of the most important pillars: exercise. And while I initially thought that this would be an easy session for me with my young body, I'm in for a disappointment. Compared to the people around me, I'm as stiff as a board, and I'm not the only one to notice. With each new movement, my somewhat bashful neighbour struggles not to laugh, until my version of the splits becomes the final straw and she roars with laughter.

After the physical workout, we're all given an iPad for a kind of IQ test. With a level of concentration you'd associate with high school exams, the group carries out a series of tasks, and it's obvious that these oldies are not computer illiterate by any means. They know their way around the tablet like a teen on TikTok, as the technology has long been an integral part of Korean culture.

The doctor who's accompanying me explains that the algorithm identifies what each person struggles with and then adjusts the programme level and intensity to achieve the best possible result. It gives both the participants themselves and the specialists, who observe from a distance, a better understanding of the programme's effectiveness and should keep everybody interested.

When my 'classmates' gather round me after our session, they confirm that that is indeed the case. 'I think everybody was very nervous at first,' says a man with a remarkably thick head of grey hair. 'It feels weird and a bit unsettling to sign up because of something "bad" that may or may not happen to you in the future, but I no longer feel that way. In fact, it has the opposite effect: it makes you a lot stronger, because you can tell you're keeping fit and you're even making progress.'

In the course of our conversation, I hear that before the programme got underway many of those taking part were quite lonely and for them the social element alone is worth it. Some have even become friends and meet up outside of sessions. But most importantly, the programme has made them all feel more in control of their lives. My neighbour, who was laughing at me earlier, captures it very well: 'Ever since childhood, you've got your path laid out for you: primary school, high school, university, work and then finally retirement. But I've been retired longer than I've attended school, without any sort of planning or support. It feels as if "life" stops as soon as you're pensioned off, as if all the years after that are merely extra time. And that's why I've long had the feeling, like so many others I've spoken to, that I just had to accept my lot and wait for what's next.' Before she resumes, she fixes me with an intense stare to see if I'm paying attention. 'I went out less and less, no longer challenged myself and became isolated when before I'd had such a bustling life. I really fizzled out, but since I've started coming here I have more energy than ever and I'm going out again to do fun things and meet people.'

Grinning from ear to ear, I say: 'I'm really glad to hear that your quality of life has improved. It's so good in fact that I'd have to attend quite a few classes to get to your level, as I just witnessed. I'd better sign up to the programme too.'

She laughs and gives me a pat on the head. 'Keeping living, my boy, that's the best medicine for ageing.' And with that she grabs her things, says goodbye to her friends and strides to the exit.

After our visit, we join a small delegation from the dementia centre for something to eat round the corner. Food is central to Korean culture and is seen as something that brings people together while doing business. As the table fills up with exquisite dishes, Hannah receives a message from Solomon: 'We've done it!'

Because South Korea is the only country in the world to have officially made dementia prevention a national priority, much of our effort in the run-up to our visit had gone into securing an appointment at the Ministry of Health and Welfare. The urgent matter of the pandemic is obviously keeping them busy, so the positive news comes as a complete surprise. But because we always dream big, we did pack our smart suits – you just never know. And now that we get to speak to the deputy minister, we're obviously glad we did.

While we were still in the Netherlands, Solomon prepared us by explaining that South Korea is a very hierarchical country. 'It's extremely important to stick to protocol, especially when you're visiting a government official. So if the invitation says: start time 9:30, the meeting will start at 9:30 sharp and not a second later.' He appears to have the gift of foresight, because when Hannah enquires when we are expected at the ministry in our Sunday best, 9:30 is indeed the designated time.

The following morning, we set off early by car for Sejong City, where most of the country's ministries are based. To ease congestion in Seoul and to spread employment and population across the nation, the construction of this administrative capital south of Seoul got underway in 2009 and officially opened in 2012. When we reach Sejong-si, it feels more like a ghost town than the bustling political heart of South Korea. An immense plain that's reminiscent of an airstrip is dotted with huge and imposing structures that rival the behemoths we saw in Moldova, and we hear the echoes reverberating among them from afar. In between these buildings are newly tarmacked roads that are all but empty, and the lack of greenery betrays the fact that the area is still under development. When she spots the surprise on our faces, Hannah says cautiously: 'As you can see, the plan to get people to move here hasn't been entirely successful yet.'

The enormous scale of the Ministry of Health and Welfare becomes apparent when we're at the entrance barriers and look up at a V-shaped white concrete bunker. Once we're past security screening, we're welcomed inside by a delegation of civil servants, who go through the questions we submitted yesterday. They clearly want to avoid any 'surprises'. After everything has been approved, we take our seats at a glossy walnut table with two crystal teacups. Hannah is standing behind and slightly to the side of the chair where the deputy minister will be sitting, so she can interpret, and behind her are the civil servants with our questions on a clipboard. We all wait for the door to open.

Just as a member of staff opens the door to the backroom and the deputy minister approaches, Jonathan, who's filming behind me, asks: 'Have you got your business card at the ready?'

The look on my face says it all. Shit, I think. One of the first things we were told before we travelled here was that when you make the famous bow you exchange business cards, and you have to hold that card with both hands. Dreading the impression I'm going to make, I rise to my feet and bow as deep as I can to compensate for the missing business card. Luckily the deputy minister is so kind as to just glance at my empty hands before he sits down in his comfortable desk chair and we start our conversation.

In response to my question why South Korea has made dementia prevention a priority, the deputy minister says: 'At present we have no cure for dementia, but the number of people with the condition in our country has risen sharply in recent years and is set to increase exponentially. That is why the government has decided to do everything in its power to prevent this, by targeting early detection of mild cognitive decline. We think we can make a huge difference by tackling the problem at the root.' He looks over to his spokesperson, who listens attentively. 'It really works. In the past, people with mild cognitive impairment would often go undiagnosed for too long and develop much more severe symptoms. As you would expect, because if nobody can tell just from looking at you and you slowly get used to the decline, there is no reason to make any changes. But if we raise awareness around this type of prevention, we can identify these people at a much earlier stage and delay or even prevent their dementia, so they can continue with the same quality of life for much longer. That is our objective.'

I'm used to politicians' fine words, but the pair of friendly eyes above the face mask lend the message a genuine feeling of compassion.

The list in front of the deputy minister doesn't leave much room for spontaneity, but when he starts reeling off figures and statistics I feel we're digressing. I decide to do something that no politician likes, least of all here: deviate from the questions. I take advantage of a brief silence to apologise and say: 'That's all very clear, but what are your own hopes for the future when it comes to dementia?'

The politician's staff talk agitatedly with our interpreter; they're not at all happy that he's being asked a personal question.

I expect the conversation to end right there and then, but the deputy minister will not be silenced. He says: 'I am glad you asked. I hope that one day there will be a cure for all forms of dementia, but until then we will focus on delay and prevention, because it can make the people who live with it happier now. Every person counts, so I hope we can help as many as possible in the future.'

The spokesperson exclaims: 'That was the last question, thank you very much!' whereupon the deputy minister gets up, bows again and brings the meeting to an end.

Soon after we board a high-speed bullet train that will take us further south. We're keen to know what national prevention looks like at community level and especially how it works in practice. In Busan, the country's second-largest city and known for its beautiful beaches and delicious seafood, Solomon has arranged a meeting with Congressman Jonghean Baek. As the region's representative, he's happy to tell us how the policy is being implemented here. As soon as we get off the train and take a taxi into town, we can see that its beauty hasn't been exaggerated. Busan feels a bit like Miami, with a coastline that curves past colourful buildings and glass skyscrapers while young and old exercise on the promenade.

A little later I'm in a coffee bar that overlooks the sea and the famous Gwangan Bridge, which has a total span of 7.4 kilometres, talking to the congressman about our experiences. I decide to ask him a personal question too: 'Why is this subject so close to your heart?'

Luckily we don't get into trouble with the assistant who's listening nearby, and the politician takes his time to answer. 'Both professionally and in my private life, I've seen the devastation that dementia can cause. So when I came across prevention in my government role, I was really keen to get involved.'

Like the deputy minister earlier, I can see he genuinely cares, and I ask: 'It's great to see how moved you are, but how do you reach people with a message that may feel irrelevant to many?'

He looks at me and pauses a moment to find the right words. 'With happiness.'

'Happiness?'

'That's right. Now that I see how much happiness prevention can bring to people, I don't feel I have to sell anything. All I have to do is share my experiences with the province, the towns and the employers. I explain to them that our prevention programme can make participants happier and will help them remain part of society for longer despite their limitations. All parties pass this on to their constituents, resulting in lots of positive responses and people coming forward to sign up.'

'That's a remarkable and very encouraging thing to hear. Thank you,' I say.

'However big or small our role may be, and however much we may have to adjust the pace of their environment to ensure these people can keep up, we see it as a shared responsibility to help them in any way we can.'

When I thank the congressman again for our candid chat, he says: 'No, this is not goodbye yet. This conversation, this meeting of cultures, calls for a celebration.'

Shortly afterwards, we sit down to the region's speciality: a sea banquet fit for a king. Jonathan and Bas salivate at the sight of the table's riches, while I tuck into my worst nightmare as graciously as I can. The guys are beside themselves with laughter as I slurp down snotty sea cucumbers, chomp on raw prawns and swallow indefinable chunks in my soup.

'Fun, isn't it, travelling with us?' Bastian exclaims before addressing the others at the table in English. 'He prefers kimchi.'

As well as scientists and politicians, we've also asked Solomon about visiting people at home. The chances of this happening had seemed even slimmer than the interview with the deputy minister, because it's rare to be invited into somebody's home in Korea, especially as a total stranger. But again, luck is on our side, because when we're walking on the beach together the next morning, Hannah gets the green light from Seoul headquarters.

Suki, a participant in the Superbrain programme, had cancelled but changed her mind after talking to her daughter. There's only one condition: it has to happen today. Hannah immediately arranges a taxi to the nearby suburb where Suki lives, which gives us a glimpse of yet another side of the country. A never-ending succession of numbered white apartment blocks in different configurations makes us feel as if we're moving through a life-sized game of Tetris. Hannah notices our surprise and again shows her versatility by filling us in. 'South Korea is very densely populated. The Seoul Capital Area alone has 24 million inhabitants, so the price of land is shockingly high. It's why there's so much vertical construction.'

We get out in front of building 506 and press the button for the 18th floor. Much of social life in Korea takes place outside the home and upon entering, it becomes clear to us just how exceptional our visit is. Suki tells us that we're the first outsiders ever to visit her here. After serving us something to drink, she immediately tells us how much weight she's lost since starting the programme and indicates her former girth.

Suki is a petite woman in her nineties with a very expressive face and great charisma. She lives alone, but to begin with her daughter joins us for moral support. She explains that her mother is very nervous, mainly because she's worried about saying something 'stupid', and may be a bit overexcited at first.

'I make sure I move every day now, starting the minute I get out of bed. First I stretch a bit, then I do my exercises, prepare a breakfast with lots of fruit, walk around the block and then it's back for a rest, because I'm not in the first flush of youth anymore,' she jokes.

If I didn't know any better, I'd think this trip was an orchestrated PR tour – everybody is so positive about dementia prevention in this country. But I know that chance and luck are the glue that hold this itinerary together, what with all the ad hoc decisions and surprises. And everyone has spoken very openly and with real joy in their eyes, so I don't doubt the positive effect of the method or the sincerity of the people I speak to.

I've noticed that when it comes to dementia, I automatically expect the worst when local or national bodies are involved. Isn't it terrible to be suspicious of positivity? But to be honest, the other thing that feeds my mistrust is the question that I've had in the back of my mind ever since we embarked on this trip: how is it possible that everybody here is so enthusiastic about dementia prevention, when it's barely even mentioned in the Netherlands? If it's so effective, then why don't we all change tack? Surely there's no reason not to if it makes both people with and without cognitive impairments so much happier?

After doing a few exercises with Suki in her living room, and getting laughed at again, she dutifully moves on to her digital homework. She asks me to take care of the flowers on her balcony: 'It brings me the greatest happiness every day. Make sure you pour the water on the soil and not the leaves, or they'll get scorched in the sun.' I follow her instructions to the letter and discover that her balcony boasts more than just a few hanging planters and is a kind of miniature botanic garden.

When we both finish our jobs we have a short rest, after which I'm the one who has to be roused. 'That's enough snoozing; it's time to get moving again,' I hear when I wake up in a daze in her armchair. After a quick and refreshing cup of white tea, we walk with Suki to the park beside her flat. The sun is low in the sky and illuminates our faces as it shines through the trees.

She links her arm in mine and starts chatting. 'My grandmother used to say: practice makes perfect. Such a powerful and simple principle. It's weird to think that it's something you forget as you get older. Aren't you supposed to grow wiser with age?' She looks at me with a twinkle in her eye. 'When you notice that you're getting better at things, it feels truly magical. It's like being young again. When I saw an improvement in my assignments, I felt so much more confident that I wanted to get better at other things too. And I can tell you that's a wonderful feeling at my age. Ninety and still wanting to improve, what's not to like?' she quips when we sit down on a rickety little bench on top of a hill.

'Look at that panorama,' I say. 'Amazing. Who says that healthy things are no fun? I, for one, will never forget this moment.'

Suki looks at me contentedly and moves a little closer to me. Together we soak in the view of the valley for a while before we walk back to her home and say goodbye.

A few days later we exchange the beautiful city on the Sea of Japan for the vertiginous capital again, where together with Team Superbrain and Hannah we work out the final part of our tour. In the next few days we want to meet the main scientists behind the programme, in the hope of learning more about its 'big secret'. Because of our earlier spur-of-the-moment meetings, some of the experts have to juggle their diaries, but in the end we manage to plan a series of visits to hospitals and universities. They're all in and around Seoul, so that remains our base.

Our first stop is Ajou University Hospital, where Professor Hong Chang-Hyung works as a researcher. He has made a huge contribution to the programme's motivational side, which is what makes Superbrain so unique. Inside the typically square-shaped hospital building, we meet him in his office, which, less typically, is filled with plants.

He launches straight into an explanation of the big difference with the original Swedish method. 'By adapting all areas of the FINGER method to Korean society, we created a kind of blueprint that we then turned into a digital programme. To this we added a sixth component, motivation. As a result, 95 percent of participants complete the entire programme.' He beams with pride. 'It's all very well to want something, but unless you're motivated you won't succeed. It's something you see in efforts to quit smoking or drinking and also in losing weight. People want to stop or live healthier lives, but they give up because the effort is in the present and the reward in the future. If they were able to see from day to day what happens to their lungs, liver or body if they persevered, I think the chances of success would be much higher. And that's exactly what we've been working on. Clarity on where you are in the programme, how much progress you're making and what your weaknesses are galvanises you and motivates you to do your best. That's the programme's big strength, and it ensures that participants keep following it, even after completion. At the end of the day, it's about achieving a structural lifestyle change and you can only do that with the right kind of motivation.'

In the same vein, one of the programme's lead doctors, Seong-Hye Choi at Inha City University Hospital, tells me that the latest research findings are even more promising. 'Our initial results were based on a 24-week programme, but we're now seeing differences in people who've been following it for a greater length of time, so we're confident that if people integrate the programme into their daily lives for longer it will be even more beneficial. Our maxim is: the longer you apply it, the bigger the benefit will be. And the greater the benefit, the less likely you are to develop a form of dementia. It's as simple as that. We're also seeing positive change in people with mild cognitive impairment in early-stage dementia: not only is the progression delayed, but the participants even manage to reverse some of the damage. So we're achieving more and more encouraging results in all areas of prevention.'

At Kyung Hee University, the very amiable Professor Yoo Kyoung Park tells us more about the role of 'superfoods' in prevention, and we learn how harmful red meat, dairy products and fried foods are. 'The next time you're at the golden arches, remember this: fried food fries your brain.' We also hear the extraordinary story of 'sticky rice'. Its growing popularity in Asia has led to an explosive rise in cardiovascular disease and in people suffering from dementia. This glutinous white rice used to be milled and polished by hand, which made it a luxury item and status symbol, but industrial methods have made it cheaper and therefore more popular.

'We have plenty of proof that an unhealthy diet is a contributing factor to disease, but luckily there's also more and more scientific evidence that healthy foods, such as those that are part of the MIND diet, can help slow the development of dementia,' the professor concludes before adding with a smile: 'I can hear you think: are all foods off limits? Of course not, and it's OK to eat unhealthy things once in a while. I'm not banning anything outright, I would just advise against it. That's a big difference. If you truly understood how much you gain by not eating it, you wouldn't even want it anymore. They're patterns and habits you need to break and replace with new ones. Once you get into that mindset, it's not difficult at all.'

Exhausted by all the information we've soaked up in the past few days we're quiet in the taxi back to the hotel, when Jonathan suddenly says: 'Tomorrow's the big day, Teun. The moment of truth.' He teases me to take the pressure off because he knows I'm finding this challenging. It's usually a pretty effective tactic, but not this time. Tomorrow I'm doing a test to see if I have a raised risk of dementia. Because the disease runs in my family – my grandmother was recently diagnosed as well – I'm more anxious about it than I'd anticipated. What worries me is not so much the thought of developing a form of dementia, because I'm not sure how I'd respond to that, but the world I'd end up in. For a long while now, I've been seeing first-hand how the current system dehumanises people, so up until yesterday I was wondering whether to go ahead, because I'm not sure if I want to know what the chances are of this fearful prospect becoming a reality. I also struggle with the increasing societal pressure for us all to have perfect lives, and I wouldn't want to change my life on the basis of a risk analysis. At the same time I'm becoming more and more confident that a better life with dementia is ours to make and that prevention plays a role in this. And that's why my curiosity wins out in the end, and I opt for a glimpse into my future.

After a night spent thinking that prevention can be a beautiful thing, but that if people do fall ill we mustn't blame them, we head to Dr So Young Moon's clinic in the morning. There's a surprising number of young people in the waiting room. I speak to a man in his late thirties who's looking after his mother with dementia and who'd like to know if he's at increased risk of developing the disease. Remarkable, I think, that it seems to be such a normal thing to check. Clearly, the belief that we can shape and control our lives has also taken root here.

When it's my turn, I'm shown a few graphs with the various stages at which dementia can be detected and what that means. The first graph isn't overly shocking: the earlier the condition is caught, the more you can do to prevent the process. The second is a lot more alarming. It shows the sudden and rapid onset of cognitive decline when it's detected too late, in which case the process is all but irreversible.

Next, the doctor gives me a brief explanation on biomarkers in the blood. These substances can be measured to see what's going on in the body and indicate whether someone has an increased risk of dementia. 'Are you ready?' she asks, as she snaps her laptop shut and gets to her feet.

'Absolutely,' I say firmly to psych myself up.

We make our way to the next room, where she takes a blood sample, thanks me for coming and assures me that the result will be in before we leave tomorrow evening. 'The good thing about this test is that it's not only a lot cheaper than an MRI, but we can also do a very quick read-out, so keep an eye on your phone.'

Still thinking about what I've just seen and heard and the role this test can play in society, I get into our taxi and shortly afterwards we walk into the Superbrain skyscraper to say goodbye to our Korean friends.

Again, Solomon is there to meet us. 'Wonderful to see you again, guys,' he says. 'Tell me, how was your trip?'

We sit down to coffee, admire the cityscape again, and then

I come out with a question that has been on my mind for days now. 'During one of our visits, I was told that dementia costs around 20,000 euros per person per year in Korea, or 200,000 over ten years. But as I understand it, your preventative approach only costs a fraction of that, about 10 percent, which could lead to huge savings in the future. So how come so few countries are looking at prevention? Doesn't every government want cheaper care and a better quality of life for its people?'

Solomon shifts to the tip of his chair. 'The healthcare ecosystem wasn't designed with healthy people in mind. Hospitals, clinics and doctors are paid per patient, so they earn more if there are more sick people. That's why prevention has received so little attention within the system. But now that society is becoming more interested in quality of life, you can see it's giving rise to a different story about healthy ageing. I'm obviously preaching to the choir, but there's a key role for prevention in all this. Once you've been diagnosed and, in the worst case, categorised as belonging to a particular group of "sick" people, it's often not just too late for yourself, but for the state as well. With all the pressure you're putting on the care system and the costs that come with it, it's all a lot more expensive for society too. So whatever your angle, prevention is always better than the cure. If we focus on that, we can not only maximise quality of life for ourselves as individuals, but also for society as a whole.'

I stand up and give him a firm handshake. 'I admire your passion, Solomon. It's great to see. If we keep trying to improve quality of life, in whatever way possible, the world will be a better place.' We hug and after walking to the table behind us Solomon returns with three gifts. 'We think it's so cool that you came all this way that as well as memories of the trip we want to give you a small present in the hope that you won't forget Korea anytime soon.'

What if I am at increased risk of dementia? What will I do? I'm staring at my new water bottle with traditional Korean motif, which gleams by my bedside in the light from the corridor. It's three in the morning and I'm wide awake, in part because my mind is still mulling over the experiences and findings from our trip, but also because my body thinks it's six in the evening. We came home three days ago, but my jetlag seems to take no notice. And I'm beginning to think that the absence of test results means a positive reading. After hearing the church bell ring strike four, I'm finally slipping into a deep sleep only to be woken by the sound of my phone shortly after.

It's Jonathan. 'Teun, I just spoke to Solomon.'

'Shoot,' I say.

'The test result came through ages ago, but it ended up in my spam...'

'Really? So?'

'Everything's fine, nothing to worry about. We'll speak tomorrow!'

Weird to think what a test like that does to you. I roll onto my left and succumb to my jetlag.

VIII Between formulaic and visionary

Pioneers of care

Belgium

When I smell oil, my eyes dart to the temperature gauge. Here we go again, I think, as the dial flicks neurotically up and down in the red zone. The message is clear: stop! Luckily, there's a big petrol station just up ahead, which saves me from a lonely wait behind the crash barrier. I adore my vintage car, a pale blue Renault Express that accommodates my housemates who use a wheelchair, but about a year ago its love for me began to wane.

After too many call outs last year I had to start paying for extra car insurance. 'If you miss me that much, just call me, okay,' a mechanic joked recently when he towed me back home in the middle of the night for a second time. In recent months, I've been doing a theatre tour based on my book *The Housemates*. With 100 performances up and down the country, I'm often driving home in the early hours. It's another collaboration with Jonathan, so he's seeing more of me than of his family and we're starting to look like an old married couple.

'Have you broken down *again*? What else is new?' I hear him laugh on the other end of the line as I lean against my car at daybreak, with the bonnet up to let the engine cool. 'Are you in Belgium?'

I check the map on my phone. 'Yes, but I've got a little ways to go yet.'

When we travel by car, we normally do it together, but not this time because he has somewhere else to go after filming.

I hear him rummage in his car. 'Send me your location. I think I'm not far from you. We'll drive in convoy, just to be on the safe side.'

After several far-flung countries, we're now embarking on a trip around Flanders to see how care for people with dementia is evolving just across the border. I'm looking forward to it, because I always feel at home here. The beautiful language, the Burgundian lifestyle and the friendly vibe in the cities never fail to cheer me up and take away any last shred of homesickness. Besides, we're visiting some remarkable homes that I've been curious about for ages. These progressive 'rest homes', as they're called over here, are managed by renowned care pioneers. We're always trying to find a balance between the range of residential facilities that a country has to offer, but with all the different government agencies it takes a while to obtain permission for the mainstream nursing homes, so they'll have to wait until later in the year.

In the course of our research, we've had mixed messages from academics, care administrators and politicians in Belgium. But the consensus was that the care system can be called complex, to say the least. The central and decentralised administrations of the different language regions are spread across the country, making the healthcare system a similarly confusing patchwork with lots of variation between care organisations.

Thankfully, today's damage is minimal, and after two hours and a bit of extra coolant my vehicle is ready to hit the road again. A little later, we turn off the motorway and drive along pretty country lanes, where I spy the odd farm through the tall wildflowers in the verge. At our next turn, however, the idyllic view is disrupted by a gigantic glass villa behind a medieval looking wall. Jonathan honks and points at the building: this must be our destination.

He'd told me we were going to an unusual place, but I've never seen such a modern and 'cool' nursing home in my life. But as I enter the car park, I do wonder how homely it's going to feel. That question is answered the minute we enter and walk across a sleek cement-look floor through large, light-filled airy spaces that feel cold.

'Welcome to Kortrijk, guys,' a carer in a dark red uniform says as soon as we enter the next living room. 'I'm Jessica, the manager. Come, let me show you to your room, so you can drop off your things.' She chuckles.

We make our way down two pristine white corridors and when we get to the end we're surprised to hear: 'This is it.' All we see is a door with a disabled bathroom sign. Amid giggling from the onlooking carers, the manager says: 'You told us you'd be prepared to sleep in a broom cupboard if necessary, so here you are.' She opens the door and points to two blue incontinence mattresses lying in the all-white space, next to the accessible toilet and seated shower with handles.

As I mentioned earlier, when we visit a nursing home we don't want to take up any room meant for residents. To stress that we're not the most demanding of visitors, we always mention the proverbial broom cupboard in preliminary interviews. The fact that we've now been allocated precisely such a space turns the metaphor into reality.

'There are no windows, so I'd advise against using the toilet just before bed,' the manager says teasingly to Jonathan, who's plumping up his pillow about two inches from the bowl.

He laughs. 'Thanks for the tip.'

Once we've settled into our 'wet room', as it's generally referred to in the care sector, I sit down to lunch. The first thing I notice are the enormous windows that make the living room look as bright and spacious as a ballroom. Directly opposite me, a young member of staff is preparing soup in the open-plan kitchen that has surfaces without raised edges (these are often used in small nursing homes to prevent people from taking anything off the counter), while the woman next to me is keeping a close eye on him and giving him the odd instruction. 'Don't forget to sauté the onion before adding it to the soup. It really enhances the flavour.' The guy is clearly enjoying the interaction. 'Of course, Mrs Lacroix, what would I do without your help?' he replies and carries on stirring the pan.

A few generously filled sandwiches later, I walk open-mouthed around the home. No endless dark corridors here, only heavenly white ones. Spread across the various floors are living rooms that are distinguished by the carers' colour-coded uniforms. And literally every time I open a door, I see the windows create sightlines throughout the building, a design that's completely new to me. All that glass makes me think I'm at the Stedelijk Museum in Amsterdam instead of a nursing home in Belgium. The director, Jan Goddaer, told us prior to our arrival that this home was designed to be 'dementia friendly', with particular attention to light.

Scientific research has shown that people feel happier and more active and alert under blue and white light. (Put simply:

candles and most lightbulbs give off yellow light, while daylight is white or blue.) During the day, this place makes the most of the abundant daylight that floods the rooms, while in the evening the light becomes warmer and yellower to help residents relax. Jan believes that this amplification of day and night is an effective antidote to sundowning, a well-known dementia symptom. Also known as late-day confusion, it refers to the increasing unrest and confusion that many people with dementia experience in the late afternoon and evening.

When we turn into the corridor behind our bathroom, I hear a rattling breath from one of the rooms. In a nursing reflex, I decide to take a look, whereupon Jonathan goes back for his camera. The door is wide open, and the nameplate by the door tells me that the person making the sound is called Jeannette. In the centre of the spacious room stands a hospital bed raised to its highest position, and the diffuse daylight filtering in through the net curtains illuminates the porcelain-hued face of a woman. The light and lonely setup instantly reminds of Eugenie's farewell, an impression that's reinforced when I come closer.

The stringy white saliva in her mouth and her rigidity suggest to me that she can barely move let alone take care of herself. When I hear her draw another laborious breath, I don't think twice and walk into her bathroom where I moisten a washcloth with tepid water. 'Hello Jeannette, so pleased to meet you. I'm visiting here,' I say as I try to make eye contact. 'Do you mind if I wet your lips to help you breathe more easily?' I show her the washcloth. Her deep brown eyes look straight through me, but she does try to move her eyelids, which tells me all I need to know. Very gently, I help her.

When her mouth is clean again, and I reach for the prayer card above her bed, I notice from the corner of my eye that it's too much for Jonathan, who stifles a sob in the crook of his arm so as not to make a sound. I gesture that it's okay if he wants to leave, but he shakes his head. I decide to read the prayer card out loud, but as soon as I see what it says I well up myself. I heave a sigh to fight back my tears, take Jeannette's hand, gently squeeze it when she glances at me and say: 'This is for you, Jeannette.' And I begin.

> Saint Rita,
>
> I turn to You with confidence, Saint Rita, patron saint of impossible, difficult and hopeless causes. Deliver me from the pain and fear that crush my spirit and grant me peace and good health. I have faith in Your mighty intercession with the Lord and have the sure hope that my prayers will be heard.
>
> Amen.

When I plant a teary-eyed kiss on Jeannette's forehead by way of goodbye, she produces a faint sound and wiggles her foot. That's the way it goes sometimes, I think to myself as I leave the room. Jonathan heads outside for some fresh air, while I sit down on the bench at the end of the corridor and mull things over. Surely this can't be described as quality of life in any way, shape or form, if you can call it life at all? Is this a dignified existence? Gasping for breath day and night, waiting for a God to deliver you? How can we speak of loving care when literally every single breath is a struggle? Where do we draw the line between humane and inhumane? Who or what are we so desperate to keep alive as family members or partners that we're willing to accept such immense suffering -doesn't it have as much to do with our own fear of mortality as anything?

'Teun, are you there?' someone asks further down the corridor.

Startled, I swallow my emotions and reply: 'Sure, I'm on the bench over here.'

A carer approaches. Judging by the colour of her uniform, she works on 'our' ward.

It's another one of those new care trends that doesn't actually solve a problem but literally gives it colourful makeover. In the care sector, uniforms always scream inequality. Thankfully, more and more people in nursing home care are beginning to catch on, but instead of changing anything it's being exploited by uniform manufacturers that say: 'So true. Why don't we make 'prettier' versions in all colours of the rainbow?' But a uniform is a uniform, whatever its shade. End of. What's wrong with 'normal' work clothing for staff? Yes, those clothes can get dirty, but so does a uniform. Both can be washed, so why the reluctance? Durability? We don't need lamb's wool sweaters or satin dresses; there are plenty of companies out there that are keen to sell their 'simple' but hard-wearing work clothing. Let's face it, at home you don't go around in uniform all day just because something might happen. Then why do we so in care? Because we think it has no effect on the residents? That we can trick them by giving the uniforms a 'homely' colour? Aren't we prioritising our own convenience over and above the happiness of people who don't have much of it in the first place?

The carer comes and stands beside me, takes one look at me and asks: 'Are you okay?'

'Thank you for asking. I was a bit sad after visiting Jeannette.'

'Oh, I know exactly what you mean. It happens to me every time I see her.' She sits down and wraps her arm around me. 'You wouldn't wish it on anyone. You know what, I'll go and sit with Jeannette for a bit. Why don't you go to the living room and have a nice bowl of hot soup. I reckon your buddy can use some of it as well.' She winks and takes me by the arm.

The next morning I wake after a surprisingly good night's sleep in our *suite sanitaire*. The smell of fresh coffee wafts in through a crack under the door. 'That's what I call a good start to the day,' I shout to make myself heard over the snoring toilet bowl. The snoring stops abruptly, whereupon Jonathan says, 'Mmm, nice', smacks his lips twice and rolls over again.

That day I have some lovely conversations with the women in our living room, talk to an informal carer who visits daily to play the piano for her husband and can't believe our luck when gold-coloured decorations are put up for a leaving do: one of the staff is retiring after forty years.

On seeing the barbecue brought out into the garden and the tables covered with snacks and alcoholic refreshments, I think: so this is all happening in-house. I think back to all those times I've been to lacklustre receptions in some hired venue where people were given a send-off with all the appropriate fanfare, but miles from the world to which they'd dedicated their heart and soul. Not so today. Here staff and residents grill prawn and satay skewers together, and everybody laughs at the tall tales told by the soon-to-be pensioner.

Jan, dressed in jeans with a flamboyant shirt and sneakers, comes and stands next to me.

'It's great that you involve the residents in this,' I say to him.

'No fuss, just all on an equal footing. That's how I like it.' He clinks his beer bottle against mine. 'You know what it is, Teun? People believe you're young at heart because you look it. But take a look around: you're not the only one, although we're often reluctant to admit it.' He beams as he watches the festive gathering. 'The reactions to this home were not measured, to say the least. It was said to be excessive, cold, too contemporary, you name it. All because of the misconception that every nursing home should look like an old man pub with doilies on the table and Andre Rieu on television. But these are people who grew up in more modern times, in the rock-'n-roll or flower-power era, who listened to Elvis, the Stones, Led Zeppelin, Pink Floyd and Frank Zappa and who may well have more liberal social and sexual mores than we do now. So who's having to adjust their idea of a traditional nursing home?' he asks, laughing.

'I must confess that I was pretty sceptical myself, Jan, and perhaps still am when it comes to the term "dementia-friendly". It emphasises the difference between people, but it also suggests that happiness can be influenced by architecture. I don't think I'm necessarily seeing happier residents here, but I do notice that the design seems to ease the agitation a bit. So far I haven't seen anyone who wants to leave or who's tugging at the door, which is all but inconceivable in other nursing homes.'

I can tell that he wants to interrupt but is too polite to do so, so I stop talking to give him the floor. 'You know, I come from the world of traditional nursing homes, and we used to see this so-called "wandering" and agitation a lot in people. But there's none of that in this home. That's to do with the architecture,' he says with conviction. 'The sightlines, which were designed especially for this building, play a crucial role in this. Wherever they are, the person with dementia can see what's going on and where to go. That instils a sense of calm, reassurance and safety. So no, it doesn't mean they're jumping for joy all day because it's so bright and the sightlines are so pretty, but if we can offer calm instead of agitation, that's a big win as far as we're concerned. Right?' he says as he takes a sip of his beer.

'I think a sense of calm and feeling safe and secure are two of the biggest markers of happiness in this phase of life, which is often uncertain, so hats off to what you're doing there. But I do think it's important to guard against using distinctive architecture to lock people up in a "novel" way, or against design becoming the overriding concern and overshadowing any sense of homeliness and warmth. It's a fine line.'

Jan nods. 'I can only raise my glass to such fine words. Cheers. To the young at heart!'

Two days later, we drive into the centre of Geel and stop outside an old townhouse half-hidden behind the big trees lining the village street. This must be Huis Perrekes.

About two-and-a-half hours north of the border with France, where Jan's home is located, is that of a woman who's become famous in Belgium for her progressive approach to dementia care, and renowned for the fighting spirit she brings to it. So a visit to care pioneer Carla Molenberghs is an absolute must during our tour around Belgium.

The contrast with the modern home we've just left couldn't be greater: the place is suffused with warmth and cosiness. Everything is made with natural materials such as wood, wool and cotton: the furniture, the kitchen, the lighting, even the art on the walls. At no point do I feel as if I'm in a rest home. When we arrive, Carla says: 'Immerse yourself. I'll speak to you later.' The stylishly dressed woman immediately touches a chord with me. Some people have charisma, and Carla is definitely one of them. Whether it's her keen eye or pleasant tone of voice, I have the impression that she understands what we're all about and trusts us to make ourselves at home here. Remarkable.

After a cup of coffee at the round cherry wood table in the middle of the living room, I'm taken on a tour by my new housemate An, who claims to have the home's 'main suite'. As I accompany her up the old granite staircase, she directs my attention to her favourite works of art to our left and right. 'That ultramarine blue tapestry may well have the most beautiful colour I've ever seen. It's so intense but hopeful at the same time. And that still life over there, that's very nicely done too.' In the two years I've spent in nursing homes, I've never heard a resident talk about the art on the walls, let alone about the ideas behind it. Much of the art I've encountered hails from a certain blue-and-yellow store, but I'm not sure if it's doing anyone any favours. Diagnosis with a form of dementia doesn't alter a person's love of beautiful things, so why do we act as if it does?

'Oh, An... What an amazing lamp, is it yours?' I ask, gazing up at the ceiling of her room, from which a thin metal frame is suspended. A vast array of ribbons forms an extravagant artwork, which looks even more beautiful at a flick of the switch.

'Mine? Oh no, kid, it was already here. It may look fancy, but it was made of old laundry from a nursing home that was shredded and given a second life as a lampshade. Not bad, eh?'

Her factual account, which strips this centrepiece of any

magic, makes me laugh. 'Sometimes it's better not to know, An. At the end of the day it's about what you see in it, not how it's made. Wouldn't you agree?'

An, who has already moved on and is in the kitchen now, quips: 'Once you know it, you can't unsee it. Whenever I switch on the light, I see the tattered frocks of elderly ladies!' She chuckles at her own observation.

An's room wouldn't look out of place in a magazine: two rattan chairs flank a brightly coloured side table and set against the wall is a pine daybed beside a dark oak cupboard. The room is also full of lush plants and the floor beside the French doors to the balcony is covered in real rugs.

Next to An's room is a smaller apartment that's occupied by a man who doesn't have dementia himself, but who lived here with his wife who did. He stayed on after his wife's death, because this had become his home too, and he's been a real asset to the household ever since. On the upper floor in the right wing, which appears to have been added at a later date, the rooms are considerably smaller but no less stylishly decorated.

After I've looked at An's kitchen, which she only uses for the odd glass of water or chilled drink, she opens another door and we find ourselves in a marble bathroom with a dusky rose bathtub, including gold taps. I can't help but joke about them: 'I thought gold taps were only ever used as a metaphor, but you actually have them?'

She frowns at her bath. 'Gold, gold... If only. "Gold-coloured" I'd say. The thing is, the marble was already here when they bought this place. Instead of erecting one of those ugly new buildings they bought this old house in the village centre and gave it a bit of a makeover, and now everybody thinks it's fancy? It's funny how things turn out.'

It makes me laugh, this cynical analysis of hers, but I'm keen to get past her scepticism. I'm curious to hear how she feels, so I decide to ask a personal question: 'What do you make of life here, An?'

She looks at me. 'It's good, kid... I feel privileged to be living here. I'm comfortable, even though this isn't my real home. The people are kind to me, the food is delicious, the house is beautiful, so I can't complain.'

I have a sneaking suspicion that she's working up to a 'but', and so I ask her outright: 'I feel as if there's something else you want to say. Am I right?'

For a moment, she seems to be in two minds. 'I don't want to come across as spoilt or ungrateful, but what I like best is real life, like you guys being here, you know what I mean? Hustle and bustle, the outside coming in. Sometimes I feel like I'm stuck on an island here.'

I'm touched by the way she opens up and gives me this incisive description of her feelings. This is something I've often spoken about in the media and now I'm hearing it from the horse's mouth. 'What you're telling me is giving me goosebumps. I know exactly what you mean. That's why I'm so glad to be spending the next couple of days with you.'

She looks up with a smile. 'A couple of days? In that case we're going to be friends.'

I extend my hand. 'Here we go, we're officially friends.'

She gives me a firm handshake.

'Shall we have another coffee to celebrate?' I ask.

An looks at me as if I'm mad. 'We just had coffee. It's time for something else.'

That afternoon, I spent some time chilling in my room, which is empty for a few days until a new resident moves in, thinking about how a few changes can make such a big difference to a space. My ceiling has beautiful wood panelling, while the white brick walls look crisp. In the corner, a forest green veneer wardrobe stands on top of vintage brown flooring, and I'm lying on a pine daybed with a burnt finish. In and of themselves, these are super simple elements made of cheap material, and yet I feel as if I'm in a Swedish boutique hotel. This is heightened by the corridors on the ground-floor with their large windows and wainscot panelling that extends into the living room. The longest corridor, with brown tiles on the floor and bright yellow paint on the walls, gives access to fifteen bedrooms and a music room for the residents. Many of the windows overlook the informal garden, which is enclosed by beautiful rustic fencing, and there are extra wide window seats from which you can enjoy the living art behind the glass.

It's great to see the ideas and feelings that were prompted by my own nursing home experience become reality. Not because I want to be right about everything, but because it fills me with hope that the changes we so badly need are possible. People often dismiss me as a dreamer, an idealist or plain naïve when I argue for a different, more homely interior with furniture and furnishings in materials that make people happy. Here in Belgium I'm staying at a home that embodies this vision, and the residents are telling me that it works. I'm pleased to be coming across such encouraging examples during our travels, so we can learn from them and together create a better future.

When it's time for afternoon tea, Jonathan picks me up and we walk over to the communal living room together. 'What do you make of it?' I ask him, knowing that he always has an unfiltered answer for me.

'It not only looks beautiful, but it feels special too. The people are alert and well cared for and make real contact. It's a nice place to be.'

As with An, I'm sure there's a 'but' coming, so I ask him straight out: 'But?'

He laughs. 'Exactly: but. It also feels a bit like a temple or a church – so peaceful and quiet. And that's a bit weird when you think about all the people living here.'

As soon as I open the living room door and the ladies at the table spot us, they start nattering. 'I'm going to sit with them,' I say. 'We'll chat more later, okay?'

Jonathan nods, positions himself close by and gets his camera ready.

The few men in this home watch from across the table as more and more ladies trickle in, sit down and keep glancing at me while talking to one another.

I think I know what they're talking about. 'Are you wondering whether I'm a boy or a girl?'

One of the residents says: 'Oh, did you overhear us?' which elicits giggling at the table.

'So, what do you think?' I ask.

A brief debate is followed by the unanimous verdict: 'Definitely a woman!' They look at me expectantly. 'Right?'

I respond by laughing: 'I'm a man, honestly.'

The women gasp in amazement.

Not much later, a young woman enters the living room and gets behind the brown baby grand. A resident called Jean jumps up from his chair and sits down next to her. He starts waving like a conductor while the pianist is still leafing through her score. I've already noticed a few times that Jean has great trouble speaking, but he's all the more expressive with his hands when he wants to communicate with the care assistants.

When the first few notes resonate through the house, many of the residents make themselves comfortable on the sofas around the piano to enjoy the music together. But three of their housemates are busy at the kitchen table, grating carrots and peeling onions and potatoes; it looks like we're eating *hutspot* (a traditional meal of mashed potatoes, carrots and onions) tonight. It's good to see that more life leads to a better life. Everything here is suffused with beauty rather than decay, and that appears to be reflected in the residents...

Just as I'm starting to nod off to the piano music, I feel a tap on my shoulder. It's Carla, who whispers in my ear: 'Now's a good moment for a chat. Let's go to my room, so we won't disturb anyone here.'

I get up and follow her.

Carla's room is right beside the front door and looks quite unusual for an office. Suspended from the ceiling is a lamp with an elegant woven cotton shade, the bookshelves are full of colourful hardbacks and to my right I see a secretary desk that seems to be made of the same wood as the bed I'm sleeping in – to my surprise, there's one pushed up against the wall in here as well.

When I ask Carla why she has a bed in her office, she answers: 'Oh, it's a rocking bed. It's the same as the one you have, but with an underframe that sways back and forth. Go on, try it.'

I take off my shoes and climb into the bed.

'The idea is that your loved ones can rock you during the final phase of your life, just as they did when you were born. So you come full circle, as it were.' Carla sits in the chair beside the bed and starts rocking me gently. 'We always hear from families that they want to do something for people who are nearing the end of their lives, but as you know that's incredibly difficult at that stage. So we came up with this bed, which both sides experience as heartwarming and a great way to connect.'

With my eyes closed, I answer: 'It's really relaxing. I feel very safe. What a beautiful design. May I ask why you do so much for people with dementia?'

She brings her head closer to the edge of the bed and says: 'Well, Teun, that's... that's...' She's struggling to find the right words, as if the answer's too big to put into words, but she's trying anyway. 'It eh... comes straight from the heart and from the very fibre of my being, every last fibre. It's a feeling beyond love. I care about these people with all my soul.' She sinks a little deeper into her chair.

'Are you afraid of being diagnosed with dementia yourself?' I ask.

There's a long pause. 'I don't know. I often ask myself that question, but I genuinely don't know... It saddens me to see people in the early stages of dementia lose their sense of self and realise that over time they'll be losing more and more. I find it hard to answer that question right now, because as with death I don't think we can really know until we actually face it. My experience has taught me that people say very different things when they're healthy than when they're not. "Just put me out of my misery when that happens," is something I hear a lot, but people don't just give up on life. I've noticed that even when someone's condition deteriorates, they still find things that make them happy. That's why right until the very end we focus on the person and never on the patient. It's an important distinction: we never stop listening to what the person wants.'

'I totally agree. But when I look at the future, I do worry

about the image that society has of people with dementia. How do you see that?'

'I really worry about that too... The worst thing is this kind of indifference, this idea of "oh, they're people with dementia, they have no idea what's going on." That lack of empathy is very worrying to me. It's seen as something that happens to other people, but it can happen to any of us,' she says with a frown. 'The measure of a society or civilisation is the way it takes care of its most vulnerable. I believe it's our mission in life to learn how to live with them as best we can.'

I conclude by asking Carla what she thinks matters most in the way we deal with people with dementia. Without hesitation she says: 'The key thing to remember is that up until the very end people with dementia have feelings and a rich inner life. They're human beings who, like you and me, look for warmth, love and security until their very last breath.' She can tell that her words have moved me. 'It's good that you're moved. Make sure you hold on to that. It's a compass that will show you the way in life.'

IX Back to the source

What community living is all about

South Africa – United States

'Would you like a piece of *boerewors*?' Arlene asks in Afrikaans, as she slides a large rolled-up sausage into sizzling hot butter.

'Yes, please,' I say to be polite and glance at Jonathan to check if I haven't made a horrible mistake. Thankfully he gives me a thumbs-up.

'Will your father be joining us?' I ask Arlene.

'Absolutely. This is his favourite dish. You better watch out that he doesn't steal it off your plate.'

We've been invited to stay with Arlene and her father David in the 'coloured' township of Fairview in Mossel Bay, where we arrived early this morning. Mossel Bay is a well-known coastal town along the even more famous South African Garden Route. The town's beautiful location between the sea and the foot of the Outeniqua Mountains makes it a popular holiday destination. But as we drove uphill towards the township, the scenery changed rapidly. The white Victorian houses made way for small sand-coloured structures with salmon-pink corrugated metal roofs, while the pleasant shopping streets with traditional verandas turned to badly paved roads and arid little playing fields.

Like Aunt Gloria, Arlene was brought to our attention by Dr Adele van Wyk, who told us that if we wanted to understand the cultural reasons why people with dementia stay at home we had to meet this woman. 'Looking after others isn't seen as a job for the state here, but as a family's shared responsibility. Not because of a lack of money, but out of love for each other,' she told us.

About six years ago, Arlene moved in with her parents, who were both showing symptoms of dementia. Her mother passed away recently, so now there's just her father David to look after and she hasn't left his side since. To ensure that Arlene has everything she needs, her brothers and sisters pay her a monthly allowance, so she's been able to leave her old job.

As the fat in the pan starts spitting even more ferociously and Arlene spreads margarine on slices of bread, her father shuffles into the kitchen. The small square table is covered with a plastic floral tablecloth, matching plates, a large mug of milky tea with the logo iDad and a bottle of chilli sauce. 'Hello boys, he says in Afrikaans, before taking two big breaths, savouring the aroma that fills the kitchen and saying: 'Ah, I thought so, my favourite fare.' He sits down.

While a simple structure, the house feels very warm and vibrant inside. Every now and then, the sun comes in through the fluttering lace curtains and illuminates David's face as he tucks into his food. It really completes the picture. The living room adjacent to the kitchen isn't much bigger than the red fabric two-seater sofa, TV and two chairs it accommodates. The front door is half open, allowing a nice, refreshing sea breeze to blow through the house.

After dinner, we help Arlene clear up, and once we've all retired to the living room together to digest our food, I ask her: 'What's it like to be caring for your parents for so long?'

'Children have to look after their parents. And not put them in a... what do you call it?'

'A nursing home?'

'Yes, one of those...'

'What do you think of nursing homes?'

Arlene looks doubtful. 'They're not bad, but they don't treat other people the way you treat your own parents. So it's better to do it yourself.'

Her father shifts in his seat and says: 'That's my daughter.'

'Yes, lovely to see you two together.'

'We like to spend time with one another,' he replies. 'That's the main thing. It's black-and-white: love will make you feel better.' He beams and looks at his daughter.

'I'm the lucky one because I get to look after my parents,' she says.

I turn to face her. 'Wow, that's amazing. I've never heard anyone in the Netherlands say that it's a privilege to look after a parent.'

'It really is. Not everyone gets the opportunity,' she says with a content look on her face and gets to her feet to give her father a cuddle.

It's nice to see that in spite of all the obstacles, reciprocity and happiness are still very much alive in this household, and that a form of dementia doesn't necessarily spell the end of a rich life.

We're given another demonstration of that the following day when we don our coats and walk with David and Arlene to the church across the road from their house. It's a square building in the same sand colour as the rest of the street. It has only a few windows and is topped with a large cross. David hasn't even crossed the threshold when he's hugged by the minister and a few other worshippers standing by the door.

'You look younger every week, David!'

David laughs and Arlene escorts him to his regular seat in a pew at the back of the church.

It makes me feel weirdly envious, which is less to do with the religious sentiment and more with the exceptional warmth I'm witnessing here. David appears to be growing happier with each gesture of appreciation, and I feel as if it's showing me something of what life is all about. Feeling seen, belonging to a community and being valued – it seems to give the people I've met during my trip around South Africa, regardless of their years or the shape they're in, a sense of legitimacy as well as a sparkle I rarely detect in my housemates. Whatever your belief system, don't you wish everybody's old age was like that?

All of a sudden, the microphone screeches into life, and the minister kicks off the service in English. 'Dear brothers and sisters, today is a special day. Brothers Jonathan and Tu... Tuin, Thun Thubes from Holland are with us, staying with our friends David and Arlene, to raise awareness of an extremely important subject. So please show them a bit of love.'

The little old organ plays the first note, a sign for everybody to jump to their feet, turn towards us and start ululating with their hands in the air.

Goosebumps!

After the service, David stays behind in the church for coffee with friends, while we walk back to the house with Arlene. I ask her: 'Do you never feel it's too much? I've heard so many stories from people and informal carers who do everything they can but are close to collapse.'

'You must be the strong one,' she says. 'When I take my father out to do something or someone comes to visit us at home, I often see him turn inward with fear and insecurity. Then it's up to me to draw him out, like he used to do with me. Step by step, over and over again. And yes, that can be very difficult, especially if it doesn't happen right away and he remains confused. I'll wait a while, watch his behaviour and have another go. I'll keep trying until I'm successful. It's a question of reading the signs and going with the flow. When people I know ask for help, I always say: "When you're always swimming upstream, you'll exhaust yourself and you won't get very far. So pay attention, dive every now and then when a wave approaches take a step back and the water will smooth out again."'

'I admire you, Arlene, I really do,' I say. We're back in her kitchen, where she puts the kettle on for instant coffee. 'Your father is lucky to have a daughter like you.'

She smiles and says, 'My pleasure.'

The next morning we set off early for the long drive to Cape Town, South Africa's Mother City, where we will be spending our final few days in a township nestled in the hills of one of the region's most beautiful spots, Hout Bay. The bay with its cobalt blue water is enclosed by steep mountain ridges, with white houses among tall trees in the foothills. It's a prime location from which to enjoy the amazing daily spectacle of the changing colours of the ocean and sky. Hangberg is situated on the lower mountain flank, which gives the raw sea wind free rein in the township's streets. For many years, it was the base of the striking looking Dr Rayne Stroebel, a fifty-something scientist sporting a long, grey-black beard, colourful clothes and a pair of trendy glasses. In our many preliminary interviews, he urged us to visit the African continent where, as he put it, 'living in the community is not a question, but the answer to what makes the best possible life. It's something I witnessed during my many years of research here and something you'll have to experience for yourself.' The main focus of Stroebel's research was the impact on people with dementia of living in the community, and his words sounded so promising that it wasn't a matter of *if* but *when* we'd be travelling here. He agreed that staying in the township overnight wasn't the best idea, so we were welcome to use his house, which is in the hills nearby.

Like Mossel Bay, Hout Bay started off as a fishing village, but due to overfishing the catches dwindled and the factories were forced to close. What little work there was for the people in the township was lost and the gap between rich and poor widened. Hout Bay is also a sanctuary for Cape Town's wealthy, who come here to enjoy one of the Western Cape's best views in 'peace and quiet'. That peace does come at a price, though, because in order to deter potential intruders from the other side of the Bay, every single house has electric fencing and warning signs provided by a private security company, whose staff wouldn't think twice about drawing their guns.

It's something I just can't get used to, as the distribution of wealth here flies in the face of all sense of justice. It makes it even more extraordinary to be accepted into the local community in a way that seems to transcend inequality and indignation. It's something we feel as soon as we arrive at a sports hall late in the afternoon, where we're met by a large delegation of women in their eighties and one man, Jeffrey.

'Welcome to the golden oldies of Hangberg,' he says, whereupon all the ladies burst out laughing. 'Our organisation is dedicated to helping the elderly, and we're honoured by your visit. All the ladies are gathering the day after tomorrow, so that should be fun.'

The building's interior is painted bright blue and features murals of children playing sports. The smell in here reminds me of my old school gym, and the props suggest to me that the hall is still being used for the activities depicted. My suspicions are confirmed when the guard at the gate admits a group of girls in leotards. 'It may be old, but the hall is still used extensively by the community. We'll let the girls get on with their dancing and I'll introduce you to some people in the township,' Jeffrey says.

The township nestles against the mountain in the shape of a half-moon, and you can tell who lives where by the different types of structures. 'Over there, high up the mountain in those darker dwellings, is where the Indians live. The Ethiopians are in the limestone huts, and a little further on, in that jumble of shacks, are the Ghanaians and the Nigerians. And "we" live here in the old centre. It seems to be getting busier and busier of late, with lots of newcomers from other countries. Who'd not want to enjoy this view?' he jokes.

As we walk down the main street and approach people in the privacy of their own homes for a chat, Dr Stroebel's picture is corroborated. 'Here in South Africa we like to look after our own, whatever the need may be. We were raised with the idea that we have to stick together,' a niece tells us. She looks after her aunt, whose memory is all but gone. 'We have coffee a couple of times a day and we do our laundry together, but what she loves the most is looking out the window in the front room. She'll wave at just about anyone walking past, so there's never a dull moment.' Next, we speak to a son who regularly drops off food for his father with dementia, and a cashier at the local supermarket who has been looking after her very elderly mother with 'forgetfulness' for three years.

Further up the hill, I hear a different story, one that's new to me in Africa. An old lady who still lives independently tells me that she worries about the influence of social media on the lives of elderly people. 'Since my children and grandchildren joined Instagram and Facebook, they often say: "See that, Mum, in Europe and America nobody looks after their parents. Everybody works. Is that how you get rich?"' She shakes her head. 'Rich? Mercedes and gold Rolexes, that's what today's youth want. In the olden days, they had to beg or steal because we had no jobs and no food, but they seem to have forgotten all about that now and look beyond our continent for examples of wealth. And yet it's right under their noses. When we no longer have each other, that's when we'll be really poor.'

It's something I haven't given any thought to here in South Africa, but it chimes with what Peter Whitehouse said to us the other week. We'll be seeing the renowned professor in the United States in a fortnight. 'Neoliberalism is the main reason behind our approach to dementia. It's capitalism on steroids. Unregulated capitalism turns individuals into consumers who just want more and more. Sometimes I'll exaggerate and say: it's almost as if human relationships come second to having the latest iPhone. But the consequences are extremely dangerous. In this never-ending obsession with "me, me, me" we forget each other and as a species become increasingly ill-equipped to deal with setbacks and challenges.'

It's poignant to be confronted with this kind of vulnerability so soon after our arrival here. In the Netherlands this culture of individualisation is rarely mentioned, neither by people working in geriatric care nor by the elderly themselves. It's almost as if we've taken this lack of societal support for granted, or we feel that by living our individualistic lives we've forfeited the right to turn to children, friends and family for some care and affection. How many times have I heard someone say: 'I don't want to be a burden on my children.' A burden? First of all, that's an assumption, and assumptions are all too often based on insecurities. Secondly: you'll never know until you ask, so have that conversation. Many people, young and old alike, struggle with a lack of purpose, focus, and meaningful relationships. I truly believe that once we've overcome our shame and we start talking, more people would come forward to look after others. At the end of the day, nobody is happy when a loved one is lonely and helpless.

Two days later I get goosebumps all over again when the hall is filled with more than forty ladies singing a cappella together. It sounds so soulful and full of passion that I believe every word, even though I don't know their language. The loving harmonies fill the enormous room with a real sense of solidarity. Then there's card playing and laughter and fresh food served from the small kitchen beside the entrance. Everybody takes the plastic bowls they've brought from home to the serving hatch to have them filled with rice and vegetables before sitting at one of the long tables.

I pull up a chair at the table with the loudest laughter, and my presence only adds to the hilarity. The topic of discussion is young men. Well, I say young. A seventy-year-old woman who lives near one of the ladies has just embarked on a relationship with a fifty-year-old man.

'Do you think that's weird?' I ask.

'You want a man, not a baby,' the lady at the head of the table says.

I laugh. A fifty-year-old baby... This is clearly a different generation.

Like the others, the woman who just spoke, Mary-Jane, wears a coarse woollen jumper under a body warmer and a beanie hat. Although the temperature outside hovers around 20 degrees Celsius, which feels very pleasant to me, it's still winter for the people here so the warm clothes stay on.

When I ask if anyone lives alone, nobody raises their hand. The youngest here are in their late seventies, the eldest is ninety-six, so you might expect some of them to live on their own, but they all have children who look after them.

'Why is that?' I ask.

'You must have someone to look after you,' Mary-Jane says firmly. 'There are a lot of elderly people who are just thrown into an old age home. And who visits?' I can hear the indignation in her voice.

'Nobody,' her neighbour says with a worried look on her face.

'Exactly, nobody. It's a sad story...'

I nod.

'Don't chuck them out of your life. They were there all your life. They were there when you needed them most. So why would you get rid of them now that they're no good? Now that they need you'

As I look at her, I realise that I feel held to account, as if she's directly addressing my generation. 'Is that what it feels like? I ask.

'Yes, I believe that a good life is a circle of shared responsibility. To maintain that circle each phase in life calls for a different contribution, but all are equally important. If the circle is broken somewhere, perhaps because people are excluded or end up on the margins of society, the entire community loses out, right?' When Mary-Jane looks around with another frown on her face, all the ladies nod.

When we finish our food, we say goodbye and leave the sports hall. Outside, the orange-red evening sun illuminates the bay and heralds our imminent departure. We drive through the township one last time, and I feel nostalgic watching the children play with old tyres and the families gather round the '*braai*' (a typical South African barbeque). I can't stop thinking about what Dr Rayne Stroebel said a year ago to persuade us to come here: 'the biggest obstacle to improving the quality of life of people in general and of people with dementia in particular is that we've forgotten about intergenerational living. But the great thing is that we can start reshaping our society tomorrow. You don't achieve real change by throwing more and more money at something, otherwise you'd all be ecstatic over there in Europe. If you want real change you'll have to convince people that it will lead to lasting happiness.'

Two weeks later, I look through my airplane window to see the same red glow illuminating the skyline of Cleveland and slowly bringing it to life. We've arrived on the fourth continent of our itinerary. Although on paper America and Africa couldn't be further apart, we're here to explore the same phenomenon: living in the community. It may not be the first thing to spring to mind in a country that's so big on self-determination and freedom, but during our preliminary research we've come across a few inspiring initiatives in the US that aim to make the future more inclusive for people with dementia.

What led us here is the question with which we always conclude our introductory meetings with researchers: 'Who do you look up to in your field?' And we would follow this by: 'Would you mind introducing us?' Not only did these tactics conjure smiles on many faces, but it also led us straight to the key figures and most relevant countries. One frequently mentioned name was that of the man we're about to meet.

Professor Peter J. Whitehouse is a professor of neurology, psychiatry, cognitive science, neuroscience and organisational behaviour at Case Western Reserve University in Cleveland. He's also a professor of medicine at the University of Toronto, a Fellow of Harris Manchester College at the University of Oxford, an author and chair of Intergenerational Schools International. But aside from this impressive track record, Peter, as I'm allowed to call him, is an incredibly kind man who's been prepared to help us from the word go. As an erstwhile key opinion leader, he was once a prominent Alzheimer expert for pharmaceutical companies the world over and consulted on the development of the first generation of Alzheimer medication. Until, that is, he suffered a crisis of conscience, because everything in that world revolved around money. As he told me in one of our first conversations: 'To me, the pharma industry came to symbolise the worst excesses of modern capitalism, with money taking precedence over people. The perverse conduct of those folks was a real eye-opener for me. I saw how they spent more money on lobbying in Washington, on lawyers to protect their intellectual property rights and on marketing to sell medicines than on actual research. There came a point when I could no longer reconcile that world with my ambition to improve the lives of people with dementia, so I decided to pursue a different path.' He subsequently began to explore special models of brain health and ageing, with a special interest in the quality of life of people with dementia. The first we heard about him – and that immediately resonated with us – was that he was the founder of the Intergenerational School. It's a regular primary school where older people, with or without cognitive challenges, work as mentors who teach social skills and, each in their own way, help foster a love of reading and maths in children. People with dementia who not only take part in daily life but even contribute to society by teaching others – I obviously had to see this for myself.

Dressed in a British trench coat and bucket hat, Peter greets us and relieves us of some of our suitcases. 'Well, here we are. It's taken two years, but at last we meet in the flesh,' he says, at which we get into a pale blue sedan and head to his house. As in South Africa, we get to stay at the professor's home, so we get to speak in a pretty informal atmosphere. As we drive across the city, he tells us all about his family and how they ended up here. In a neighbourhood that goes well with his outfit, we park on the drive of a house that wouldn't look out of place in the English countryside. 'We love the architecture of this big home. It may seem fancy, but it's just as old inside as it looks from the outside, you know,' Peter says laughing. 'Come in, my wife's been baking, so let's have tea.'

'Did you sleep well?' It's early the following morning and there's another selection of freshly baked treats in front of us.

'Very well, but I can't wait to see your school.'

Peter laughs. 'Great, I like it. Raring to go.'

I've been looking forward to this meeting for years, so I can't pass up this opportunity to chat. 'I have so many questions for you. May I ask you some over breakfast?'

Peter laughs even louder. 'Of course, fire away.'

'How do you see dementia?'

'Dementia is a label that divides people and doctors,' he says cautiously. 'The danger is that once a label has been applied it's rarely questioned. But what we often fail to realise is that labels change over time. That's important to remember when we say that something is just the way it is. Perhaps the best example is the label that goes with the best-known form of dementia, which came about by accident.'

On 3 November 1906 Alois Alzheimer, a clinical psychiatrist and neuropathologist, presented a case of 'a peculiar severe disease process of the cerebral cortex' at the 37th Meeting of the Southwest German Psychiatrists in Tübingen. He described a woman in her fifties who suffered from paranoia, progressive sleep and memory disorders, aggression and confusion. Alzheimer had observed her for five years until her death, and his report listed prominent plaques and neurofibrillary tangles in the histology of the brain. The presentation provoked little interest, despite an enthusiastic response from fellow psychiatrist Kraepelin, who included 'Alzheimer's Disease' in an edition of *Psychiatry*, which was an influential publication.

'So the disease was effectively created when a colleague and friend created a classification on the basis of Alzheimer's findings, which then led to research into this new "Alzheimer's Disease". To begin with, it was a label for young people with this specific form of progressive cognitive decline, before it became a label for everyone, regardless of age, with the same symptoms. Next, it came to encompass "mild cognitive impairment", followed by "early mild cognitive impairment". And now it even includes "subjective cognitive impairment". If we're not careful, we'll end up giving everybody preventative treatment. It's a case of disease mongering or diagnostic creep, of the threshold for diagnosis becoming lower and lower. I'm exaggerating a bit to get my point across, but it does create the impression that we want everybody to have an illness so we can treat them. I don't think that's helpful. In fact, we ought to accept some aspects of life as we age and not medicalise or label them.'

It's obvious that Peter also likes to make the most of an opportunity to chat. He takes a sip of coffee from his mug and quickly resumes.

'The danger, as with dementia, is that a label leads to stigmatisation. And when that happens the person in question will deteriorate fast. A label is used to say that someone is different and that we don't want anything to do with him or her because we're scared of turning into them. That's what makes a stigma so dangerous. It dehumanises. Our national Alzheimer's Association is a case in point. They create a lot of fear by saying: "Dementia is more dangerous than cancer. It's worse than death, the worst thing that can happen to you. That's why we must treat everybody who has it as a special subset and invest even more money in solving the problem." To no avail, because we'll never find one single "remedy",' Peter says with conviction.

'Doctors and scientists often raise false hopes. Even the current chair of the World Dementia Council, the world's leading agency in the field of dementia, tells the media that it's only a matter of time before we have a cure. As does our own Dutch Alzheimer's Association, which claims that we'll get there in 2025. But in reality we're not even close to a cure. Mainly because there's more and more evidence that Alzheimer's isn't just a single disease with a single cause – that's a myth. So how many cures will we need? Besides, the symptoms are closely related to ageing; are we implicitly trying to cure ageing too? The fact is, as we grow older our abilities decline, so perhaps we shouldn't brand everything a loss, but look at what older generations can contribute in terms of experience, wisdom, etc. Like we did in the olden days. When we view ageing as a collection of ailments that must all be cured so we can achieve eternal life, we end up writing off an entire life stage. That doesn't reflect reality in any way and only undermines the happiness of a lot of people.'

'Wow,' I say. 'And that was only one question.'

Peter laughs again. 'It's an occupational hazard. I do go on a bit sometimes.'

'It's great to see that after all these years you're still so passionate about what you do. Very inspiring.'

His wife, Dr Catherine Whitehouse, comes in and says: 'Time to go, guys. The school's about to open and they're expecting you.' Catherine is a psychologist and she's the one who came up with the idea of the Intergenerational School and then developed it together with her husband.

The school is in a palatial building that puts me in mind of *The Crown*. 'This used to be a hospital, but now it houses senior living apartments, a nursing facility and our school. We couldn't wish for a better location,' Peter says as we enter. All thoughts of castles disappear as we walk down the corridors, where jackets hang on coat hooks outside the classrooms.

When Peter is talked to by someone he knows, a young man in his thirties comes up to me. 'Nice to meet you. I'm Greg, the school principal.' When I look surprised, he smiles. 'No worries, I always get that. People expect a principal to be a wise old man, but some of us are a bit younger, you know.' He laughs.

We walk down the corridor and chat about the school.

'Look, here's my office,' Greg says at the bottom of the big central staircase and points to a room with an old Obama election poster on the wall. 'He's always been a huge inspiration to me as a young black man, and that's helped me get to where I am today.'

'That's great to hear,' I say. 'Did you always dream of doing this?'

'This? No, are you crazy! It never even crossed my mind, until I landed a good job after college and came back to my old neighbourhood. Suddenly I was seen as a role model, and that made me want to create a place where children would get the same opportunities that I had. That's how I ended up here. This is a public school in an area where a lot of kids grow up in poverty and start life at a big disadvantage. Our method of teaching, which gives our students a safe place to learn, healthy food and support in any way we can, has turned that into an advantage.'

'Really? How does it work?' I ask.

'As any educator will tell you: relationships are the key to success. Children come in at the age of four when all they know is their family, so to make sure they thrive and flourish we have to create a family. We do that by adopting a certain attitude as a team, but more importantly we have mentors who complete our vision. Sure, we can give children books, but to bring that material to life it needs to be tailored to the community and that's what we do here. We believe that you learn best in a social setting. You'll get to see that in practice in a minute, because I think Paul's waiting for you.'

When I thank Greg for his fine words and leave the office, I see Peter approach with a man who's roughly the same age as he is. 'You must be Paul,' I say. It's him.

Paul, dressed in a pair of brown trousers, a shirt and burgundy sweater vest, is retired and frequently visits the school as a student mentor. He can come in when he feels like it; he has no obligation to do so. 'We'd better hurry,' he says. 'My student Charlotte is waiting for us in Miss Megan's class. Normally there's no rush, but because you're here, I agreed with the teacher yesterday that we'd stop by before phys ed and that starts in just under an hour.'

Charlotte seems to be expecting him, because the moment we walk in she jumps up and runs over. Paul beams when he gets a big cuddle, and then the two of them find a place where they can do some sums. Charlotte, an eight-year-old girl in a leopard-print T-shirt and her hair in two top knots, sits down cross-legged and relaxed on a grey bench at the end of the corridor. Peter and I watch from a distance.

Paul asks, 'How much is this?' and shows her a maths worksheet with sums.

'Fourteen,' Charlotte replies immediately.

'And this?'

'Eleven,' is the equally fast answer.

After about thirty minutes of language and maths games, a classmate comes to collect Charlotte so she can get ready for gym class. But first she gives Paul another cuddle. After she's left, I sit down next to Paul on the bench and ask him why he decided to become a mentor at this school.

'My whole life I worked hard, and when I retired I really wanted to do something meaningful. I wanted to find a new purpose and I found it here.'

'I don't really need to ask, because I can see you're beaming, but how does it make you feel?'

All of a sudden, Paul bursts into tears. 'It's very fulfilling for me. They appreciate it... I don't have any children of my own... I'm glad to do it.'

It's amazing to witness the power of inclusion up close, and to see the effect on people when ageing isn't viewed as a loss but as a benefit to society. The school administration doesn't specify which of the mentors have cognitive challenges to make sure that the person entering the classroom isn't immediately given a label. 'It doesn't add anything to the lessons let alone to the relationship that develops between mentor and student,' Greg explained when I asked him about it. This is quite a contrast with the Netherlands, where a dementia diagnosis is your entry ticket to everything 'care' related. And in our country an initiative like this would only be for people with dementia, while its strength actually lies in diversity.

After Paul has left, Peter joins me on the bench and asks: 'So what do you think?'

'I'm touched to see how much these moments mean to Paul. It's truly special. It was the same in Africa. Those moments of solidarity, when people felt they belonged and mattered, made a huge impression on me. It's a powerful antidote to the loneliness and despair that I often see in my housemates. It makes me wish that we could integrate this sense of community into the care system. Surely, there must be a way?'

Peter nods. 'Absolutely. Before we had nursing homes, people were basically cared for in the community. And we're going to have to go back to that, to normalise and to humanise people, that we have made abnormal and made inhuman, because we have given them a label and said "because you have this label, you belong in an institution". If we can just shift people's attitudes and say, "The real answer here is friendlier communities", then friendlier communities will help us all in the future. We will create happier lives for all of us, not just people with dementia.'

X A different outlook, a different outcome

Taking control of your happiness

Twello, the Netherlands

As the bleating of sheep gets louder, I roll over on my camp bed in the conservatory and look through the window to see the area shrouded in thick fog. We've spent the past two days in a home with a long history, Huize Hunderen. Dating back to the seventeenth century, the whitewashed, two-storey country house is set in lush green grounds and surrounded by a moat.

Not the most obvious location for a nursing home, but that only makes it more interesting. We're here to have a look at the other end of the care spectrum. Over the past two-and-a-half years, people at the organisations we visited would often say: 'I bet you go to private facilities for positive examples? That's too easy. Anyone can provide good care when money isn't an object.' But is that really true? We've seen so much excellent care in places where people had little money to spend that we felt compelled to investigate whether more affluent institutions are able to achieve the same.

There are two organisational structures in Dutch nursing home care. Mainstream care and private care. The latter has boomed in recent years. The main difference between them is their legal status. Mainstream institutions are foundations, not-for-profit organisations (which is not to say that they make no profit) that rely on the government and the statutory contributions of residents for their funding. Private facilities are for the most part limited companies, and often subsidiaries of listed businesses that do set out to make a profit. In the Netherlands, private institutions receive the same amount of government subsidy as mainstream nursing homes, for instance in the form of money linked to a particular care indication, but are free to charge residents more. This has earned them a great deal of criticism. 'Making money at the expense of the elderly, how dare they?' and 'Private care is destroying mainstream care, so in the future only the rich will be able to afford care' – I've heard it a million times in my still young career, and the gap between the two organisational types appears to be wider than ever.

The private sector gets most of the blame for the widening gap: it's thought to want to take over rivals left, right and centre, lure staff from mainstream homes and cut corners when it comes to providing care, because the facilities are run as businesses. But there's another way of looking at it. I'm not an economist, but the basic knowledge I have tells me that the 'free market' is driven by supply and demand. In this case, demand is huge and will have to be met one way or another. Private care will be a lot more expensive, that's true, but is that really an issue when some people are prepared to pay a bit more? People are free to choose, right?

In short, it's high time to start making sense of the 'war' between mainstream and private care. And where better to start than in the stronghold of the 'arch enemy' itself?

Huize Hunderen is run by Wonen bij September, a private care provider that has expanded rapidly in recent years and is known to many for its high-quality care for people with dementia. The organisation encompasses multiple brands, each with its own 'identity', and claims to cater to all the different profiles in the Netherlands. So if it's luxury you're after in old age, that's an option, and if you're on a state pension you're welcome in one of the less lavish homes.

When, a little later, the relentless bleating has driven me out of bed and I'm sauntering around the 'castle' in my underwear, en route to the shower, I'm accosted by one of the residents. 'Hello, young man, look at you all starkers. Shouldn't you be wearing a dressing gown?' Anneke is a vibrant woman in her eighties, and you can tell just by looking at her that she's had a good life.

'No, I'm fine, Anneke. I'm on my way to the shower.'

'Ah, I see... that explains a lot. I won't keep you then.'

'Anytime, Anneke. I'll see you for coffee in a bit, okay? Or are you going into the village?' I'm walking and talking at the same time and turn to catch her answer.

'That's right. I'm heading into Twello in a moment, but I'll pick up something nice for afternoon tea. How does that sound?'

'Delicious!' I say and enter the bathroom.

If you're thinking 'how sweet of him to play along' then you're wrong. Anneke really walks the two-and-a-half kilometres to her favourite shops by herself several times a week. It was agreed in consultation with her family, who also sanctioned a bank card for 'mama', so she can make her own purchases. It's something that makes me happy, because how great is it to be free to do as you please despite a dementia diagnosis?

And she's not walking down some quiet little footpath either. To get to the centre of the village, Anneke has to first cross a busy country lane, with cars and tractors whizzing past. Next, she has to traverse a dual carriageway, a trunk road connecting Apeldoorn and Deventer, followed by a railway line. There's plenty of opportunity for tripping, getting lost, misjudging situations and getting run over. 'It comes with the territory,' her daughter said. 'Mama has had an unconventional and outgoing life, so we owe it to her to find ways of maintaining that lifestyle for as long and as best as we can.'

The principle of someone having their own money is commendable too, because if I had a penny for every single time Ad looked disappointed when we were in a shop and he couldn't buy me anything. 'Sorry, lad, I'm afraid I have no cash on me,' he always says. I can't stress this enough, but people with dementia aren't crazy. Do they act weird at times? Sure. But that doesn't mean they automatically forget everything they've spent a lifetime doing, such as buying and paying for groceries. What makes it even easier these days is that my housemates don't have to remember a PIN for contactless payments. Just set an upper limit and you allow someone to literally buy a sense of dignity...

Here it's helpful that the village shopkeepers have agreed with the nursing home that if Anneke buys multiples of something the items can be returned, no questions asked. Obviously, that doesn't apply to the butcher's and the baker's, which Anneke is only too aware of. But I can hear the voices of the doom-mongers in my head: 'Nice, but you can really only do that in a village.' How's that? Every town or city has neighbourhoods that operate in much the same way as a village. One of my best friends comes from Twente, a fairly rural area, and has been living in Amsterdam Oud-West for years. He says that he's never felt more 'village-y' and rarely leaves the neighbourhood.

Of course it helps if people are familiar with the region, town or locale. If you'd lived in the centre of Rotterdam for much of your life and then moved to a nursing home in the countryside around Maastricht, in the far south of the country, it would take you a while to settle and get to know the area. But even then: is that a reason not to try?

After a refreshing shower, I join my regular posse for breakfast. On my left sits Truus, who loves to read gossip magazines and spends the rest of the time drawing, opposite me Rinske, who's always full of smiles whatever the ladies at the table say, and to my right the life and soul of the party, Marjolein, who asks: 'So tell me, are you getting used to this place?'

'I'm still a bit gobsmacked,' I answer.

'Really, why is that?'

'Well, it's so beautiful and spacious here. I'm not used to that.'

Marjolein looks delighted. 'That's nice to hear, because I felt exactly the same when I arrived here. I'm from a rural backwater, so to end up here, with all these antiques, the sheep in the meadow and that view... We're lucky to be living here, and I know it.' She tops her bread with *vruchtenhagel*, fruit-flavoured sprinkles. 'When we finish our sandwiches, I'll take you to my favourite spot, the biggest Japanese nut tree you've ever seen. It's magnificent, isn't it Rinske?'

'Yes, the *Ginkgo biloba* is gorgeous, Marjolein,' Rinske says firmly.

Huize Hunderen is made up of the main house and a coach house and has a total of nineteen apartments. Most of the people with more limited mobility are in the coach house, because it's lower and has a more practical layout. I'm sleeping in the conservatory behind the living room in the main building, which gives me a lovely view through the tall windows of the moat and the rear of the estate. During the week, the conservatory is used as a 'gym' for gentle exercise and at the weekend it's a kind of cultural platform for piano concerts and other forms of art. Much of the interior has been kept in its original state, so that when you walk around the house it breathes, groans and creaks ever so charmingly. Thick red curtains absorb the sound that ricochets off the ornate ceilings, and the old armchairs with matching side tables create the impression that 'the lady of the house' could make an appearance at any moment.

After helping clear the breakfast table, I hang around in the kitchen for a while for a chat with José, the manager, and I tell her that I'm meeting the home's founder later. 'I'm sure you'll get on well,' she says.

'Really? Why?'

'Michiel's background is not in care but in civil engineering, so he doesn't give a hoot about sacred cows, which is very refreshing.'

'That bodes well,' I say before asking the question I ask everywhere I go – and which usually gets a negative response: 'Would you want to live here yourself?'

'Oh yes. I'd move in tomorrow! And I'm not saying that because I'm the manager. I don't think you could work here if you didn't feel that way. I tell all the people on the floor: "Try and work with the residents to make this their best day possible. That's what matters." I don't have to check up on them to make sure they're sticking to the timetable. Everyone's going to get their medication on time, that goes without saying, but everything else comes second to the residents' happiness. That's what they're here for, and it's our job to make that happen. It's their home, and we're here to provide some entertainment or, if they prefer, peace and quiet. Simple as.'

'Nice! And do you have the freedom to do that?'

'More than enough, and luckily we have a lovely bunch of employees who feel the same way. That's what you need to do things differently. Trust. Michiel gives me that trust, and I give it to the people who work here. Look, there he is.' José points to the drive, where a vintage BMW has just pulled up.

Out of the impressive car comes a smart looking man in his forties, wearing white trainers, jeans and a woollen jumper over his shirt. A successful dude, I think to myself.

Michiel and I decide to go for a stroll around the grounds and launch straight into a discussion about the battle between the different worlds of care. I can tell from his face that he's up for a sparring match.

'With an entrance like that you don't exactly debunk the image people have of private care,' I tease him.

Michiel laughs. 'Rightly so, because I'm not the one who should adjust his image; it's the people who say that. As one of the wisest men in history once proclaimed: "Ignorance is the root of all evil." I don't know if it's the root of *all* evil, without wanting to cast doubt on Socrates, but I think it's definitely the greatest contributing factor. What we don't know is scary. It's easy to judge and even easier to condemn. That's the thing about ignorance: when you're not familiar with something, it doesn't affect you either. I'm super proud of all our eighty establishments and the great staff that work in them. So hit me, Teun, what else have you got for me?'

It's obvious that we click, and it's nice to be able to talk openly. 'My social conscience is telling me to ask you this: is it really possible for someone who's been in rental accommodation their whole life and who hasn't built up any equity and therefore has very limited means to live in one of your facilities?'

'Absolutely,' Michiel replies. 'That's another misconception. Look, right now we're in the most upmarket building, but we have multiple brands of which *Dagelijks Leven* is the biggest. They manage fifty of the eighty homes, and they're all accessible to people on a state pension. And everybody eats the same things. So the reason why people sometimes pay more is simply down to location. We like to supply a demand, the same as in society at large, but the vision and the quality of care are identical across the board.'

Once we've crossed the wooden bridge over the moat and sit down on two bistro chairs in front of the house, I say to Michiel: 'I agree, the funny thing is that when you arrive here, you think, wow, look at this fancy castle, it must be very swish, but I don't feel that that's what this place is all about. It must be wonderful to live in these surroundings, don't get me wrong, but it's not the luxury that creates the quality of life. It's the kindness with which the staff interact with the residents, more than anything. And that doesn't cost a penny. You're given the space to live here. People walk in and out, and when I woke up to the sound of sheep this morning, I noticed a cat at the end of my bed. That's unheard of in my nursing home.'

Michiel is lifted by my words. 'Private or mainstream, it's irrelevant. The real question is: what do people with dementia need to have a nice day? That's the starting point. If there's a garden you can look at but not walk in, and you don't have the mental capacity to understand why that's not allowed, then that creates confusion. So we need to look at how we can get people to go out and walk around in it. Luckily, there are plenty of mainstream facilities that offer excellent care and unfortunately also private institutions doing a bad job. It's not about the money, but about the vision.'

'May I sit with you?' asks Harry, who's heading towards us with his rollator.

'Of course,' Michiel says. 'We're having a nice chat, so please join in.'

Once I've helped Harry light his cigarette, he looks around contentedly and says: 'Nice spot you've picked.'

I turn to Michiel again. 'Let me play devil's advocate for a minute. I see you have a lot more staff than other places. Doesn't that make it much easier to provide personalised care?'

His eyes are ablaze as he speaks. 'I notice that the "dichotomy" really gets to me, because I want to help people. That this is something that puts food on the table is fine as long as you're transparent about it. Earning money from care is seen as almost dirty in the Netherlands, but that's unfair, because state-funded facilities make profit too. Some of them spend a whopping 40 percent on overheads – that's to say: on management – while we're making do with 10 percent. That enables us to organise things differently and to have many more care assistants on the floor. So again, it's a question of having a vision that leads to better management.

It strikes me as strange that the Dutch feel more comfortable with a state-funded organisation that makes a profit and spends 40 percent of it on overheads than with a privately run company that does the same but with overheads of only 10 percent so there's more money to provide better care. So we'd rather see tax revenue misspent than organisations backed by private investors achieving similar returns.

The Netherlands spends 18 billion euros a year on nursing care. So if we take a different approach and cut the overheads from 40 or 35 to 10 to start with, we can reduce that figure by 25 to 30 percent. I say: let's do that! Think how many more staff we'd be able to hire with that. Surely we ought to stop pouring money into a system that isn't working and very few people want to live in? Especially when you think that in the next 20 years more people will need care, but there'll be less money available. I'd like to invite state-funded care executives to sit down with us and look at how we can organise things more efficiently or wisely while at the same time delivering higher quality care. Better care at the same price, what's not to like?'

'That sounds almost too good to be true. Can we really cut that much on overheads and levels of management?' I ask. 'I doubt that your 10 percent pays for the same number of people as the 40 percent in mainstream care?'

'It's definitely possible, but let me clear up another misconception first. We don't pay our staff more than the mainstream care sector does, and we don't have a bonus system or anything like that either. Again, what we achieve owes more to our vision and how it's implemented. My colleagues on the floor are doing the work every day and they know how to provide good care, so if I were to interfere with that things would go wrong. I have to trust them and give them the space they need.

The mainstream care sector has more managers and more management levels that don't add much and sometimes even get in the way. We ought to have the courage to question how much they all contribute to the residents' happiness. If the bottom line says it doesn't amount to much, those people and the money are better deployed elsewhere. The fundamental difference in our organisation is that the residential staff are in charge. That's not to say that we come running the minute they snap their fingers and accommodate their every wish, but we do try to make their job as easy and enjoyable as possible. The mainstream care sector could take a leaf out of our book, but it demands a lot from managers and administrators. It forces us to re-evaluate current roles and become better at facilitating.

I hope we can end the ignorance surrounding the differences in care and push each other to change the care landscape for the better. I'm convinced it can be done.'

'So am I,' Harry says, whereupon all three of us burst out laughing.

'I really enjoyed our conversation, Michiel', I say.

'You build bridges. That's really inspiring. We need many more unifying voices in the care sector, and fewer people who keep over-egging the differences, that much is clear to me. Thank you very much.'

We give each other a firm handshake and with that he gets back into his classic car. And as Harry and I wave him off, he slowly disappears from view.

An hour later I'm sitting next to Rinske and Marjolein, watching Andre Rieu, who's also made it into this little castle, when I suddenly hear a 'Hello young man' behind me.

I turn my head.

'I promised you something, didn't I?' It's Anneke, standing in the doorway with a small bag of chocolates.

'So you did, Anneke,' I say without letting on that it had slipped my mind. 'Did you have a nice time in the village?'

'It was a pleasant walk, more than anything. It always does me good. Would you like to come to my room? I'll bring a pot of tea.'

Shortly afterwards, Anneke welcomes me in by saying:

'Make yourself at home and feel free to have a nosey; there's plenty to see.'

It's a spacious room that overlooks the beautiful grounds and that's full of antique furniture. The deep-pile carpet on the floor goes well with the thick fabric curtains. But what really stands out is all the art.

'Wow, look at these amazing artworks.' Everywhere I look, I see colourful paintings in all sizes, small busts as well as sketches underneath a half-empty wine glass. 'You're like a proper artist here in your own studio,' I say as she stops in front of one of the paintings and studies it closely.

'I'm an okay painter, even if I say so myself, but I used to have a job buying art for office buildings. That meant I always knew interesting people, like the man who did that piece over there. Karel Appel himself gave it to me. Oh, the parties I went to with him.' Her cheeks flush. 'Yes, I've had a good life. It was very rewarding.'

'Was?' I ask. 'How about now?'

'Oh, what can I say? My life is like the painting I did this week.' She picks up a small canvas, which is lying on her desk next to a photo of her late husband. It's a simple landscape in watercolour, with trees lining a path that narrows as it inches towards the horizon before vanishing around the corner. 'Look, I love nature and trees and beautiful skies with clouds that are always moving, because that's what I'm like too. And life begins broad like this path and narrows as you get older, until you reach the vanishing point.'

'What a lovely analogy,' I say.

Anneke beams.

'You say that life is narrowing. Where on the path would you say you are right now?'

Anneke looks at her work again and says: 'Well, we never

know, do we, but I'm eighty, so I'm sure it won't be long before I reach the end of the road. But until then I'll keep doing what I want, even though I have to beg and bargain a bit more in here than I was used to.'

'Yes, you strike me as a free spirit,' I say.

'Absolutely. I don't like to be told what to do. That can be pretty annoying for the staff, but I always pick up some flowers in the village to make it up to them.

And with that she throws me a mischievous look that makes us both smile.

An ordinary paradise

Mariahout, the Netherlands

'It's as if we're moving around Anneke's painting,' Jonathan remarks a week later when we're walking with a group of people in the province of Noord Brabant.

I see that the path ahead does indeed stretch all the way to the horizon and smile. Knotted willows line it on either side, their branches, like the clouds above, constantly in motion. When we arrived at Grootenhout we were told to keep our coats on so we could head straight out for a stroll with the residents. Not through the garden, but in the woods behind the estate.

Although the name evokes a similar kind of place, this isn't anything like our previous location. It reminds me of the rural area where I grew up. Grootenhout is made up of several care farms, scattered across neighbouring villages. With their beautiful tumbled bricks and vivid doors and shutters, they appear to be straight out of the Burgundy region.

The story of Grootenhout starts with an inspirational couple, Noudje (a veterinarian) and Doris (an estate agent), who were caring for his mother who had dementia. They were baffled by the care that was offered to people with the condition, so when Noudje's mother's health deteriorated they decided to care for her full-time. 'What we saw in nursing homes was nothing like the life we were used to round here. There had to be another way,' Doris said during our preliminary interview, which took place at their very first care farm in Mariahout. Noudje: 'We didn't let our lack of knowledge get in the way of making my mother's life as comfortable as possible, and as time went by we were starting to wonder if we might want to look after other people in this way. So then we thought: let's do it! Now that we have several more farms, it still feels as good as it did in the beginning. Life here with us is as "ordinary" as it can be, and people think that's remarkable... Does that make sense to you?' Laughing, Doris adds: 'So if you'd like to see a normal home, you're very welcome to stay with us.'

During the stroll, I walk beside Wil, who doesn't look up at the trees but down at my silver-coloured sneakers. Every three steps, she exclaims: 'Look at that, beautiful!' Dementia can lead to disinhibition, which is associated with loss of decorum and a wide spectrum of behaviours, including extreme anger, sadness or fear, or in Wil's case excessive cheerfulness. 'Blooming Nora, how cute!' she says when the dog owned by fellow resident Hans trots past.

In countries where dementia is less well-known, such disinhibition often makes people feel ashamed of their parents or loved ones. As a result, not everybody had the courage to take part in our research, however much they would have liked to. People feared being judged by the community, especially in places with a less liberal attitude to sex and social mores. The entire family's honour could be at stake if outsiders saw anything improper. It was heartbreaking to see that it wasn't so much their parents' behaviour that caused them pain, but the stigma attached to it. It doesn't have to be that way, if you ask me. Such symptoms are caused by a condition and are nobody's fault. So I'm pleased to see that Wil's daughter Irene, who has come along on today's walk, seems comfortable with her mother's behaviour.

When we emerge from the woods, we get a better sense of the care farm's layout. First we walk past several paddocks and the riding school's stables, where residents can often be found looking after the animals. Across from the big paddock are six wooden cottages with a Hansel and Gretel vibe. They make me think of luxury holiday homes. Behind these dwellings is a small courtyard with some more houses. To the right of the main farmhouse, Grootenhout I, where people eat and do activities, are a further two paddocks and beyond them another house and a large barn with a workshop for the residents and a proper hairdressing salon.

Besides the lively atmosphere at the care farm, I'm struck by the fact that none of the roughly twenty people who have come on this walk use a wheelchair. That's unique, to say the least, because at my nursing home the ratio is totally different, with nine out of fourteen people permanently confined to wheelchairs. It makes me wonder: is this a matter of selection at the gate or the outcome of visionary care? The former would really trouble me, because you'd be giving preferential treatment when it's actually those who are less mobile who could do with a bit of help in getting fresh air. But if it's down to vision it's bordering on revolutionary, because both at home and abroad people with dementia are seen as mainly apathetic.

Shortly after we enter Grootenhout l, the wood burner is lit in the communal living room that wouldn't look out of place in an urban cafe with its stylish jumble of chairs, sofas and carpets. Big pans on the dining table give off the unmistakable aroma of *boerenkool* (a traditional potato and curly kale dish) and bacon.

'I hope you guys are hungry,' says a woman who puts down some pickles to go with the mashed potato dish.

'You bet, especially after that delightful walk,' I say. 'May I ask who you are? Does your mother live here, or are you a volunteer perhaps?'

She laughs. 'How silly of me. I'm supposed to introduce myself to new people, but I've seen so much of you on social media that I feel as if we've known each other for ages. My name is Anja, and I'm a band 5 nurse.' (That's another healthcare affliction in the Netherlands: always including your level of training in introductions.)

'Your civilian clothing confused me,' I remark cheerfully. 'Are you free to choose what to wear?'

'Yes, that's an important part of the philosophy here. Equality is at the forefront of everything we do, and that doesn't change just because you have a diagnosis. That's why we work in our own clobber.'

You see, I think to myself, it's a question of just doing it. No ifs and buts. Now I literally can't distinguish between visitors and residents. 'Great.'

After two big plates of *boerenkool* with everything (gherkins, silverskin onions, mustard, crispy bacon pieces, a splash of vinegar and Dutch smoked sausage), we take our bags to the guest room in Grootenhout III, the house opposite the main building. When we get there, the residents wave at us and we're met by one of my very first 'care friends', Francien van de Ven, who's the manager here and one of the people behind the vision. This proud Brabant native is in her forties and fairly petite, making her distinctive glasses and smile look even bigger than they are. Every time I speak to her, I strongly feel that the staff shortage in care would be resolved overnight if half of all workers were more like Francien. Her upbeat, driven, empathic and can-do attitude strengthens my belief that the real power of care is in the hands of those who provide it...

'How wonderful to see my boys again!' As I mentioned earlier, Francien was the one who introduced Jonathan and me. Since then, she's been a font of knowledge for our research and travels. 'Did you really have to go all around the world before coming here?' she teases us. 'And by the way, Teun... you two are sleeping in the room of our nightshift worker. He's off sick, so I thought that since you're a trained nurse you might want to step up to the plate?'

I laugh out loud. 'You're on it, as usual. You don't see problems, only solutions. Of course I'll do that for you.'

I've spent a lot of time on the phone to Francien and I briefly visited the estate before, but I haven't yet had a chance to experience the 'real life' that this organisation is known for. It's why this was one of the go-to destinations on our tour.

As my neighbour Wilma leads the way up the stairs to show me to my room, I ask Francien, who's following behind: 'I need to ask: how come I haven't seen anyone in a wheelchair yet? Everybody waves, people walk up the stairs unaided... Do you select at the gate?'

'I'm glad you mention it, I really am,' she says. 'It's a common reproach, so I welcome the chance to rectify it.' She puts my suitcase on the bed and stands beside me. 'We don't have apathetic residents here, but people who react when someone enters, and that sets us apart from big institutions where you see a lot of folk asleep with their head on the table. If you've worked in that system for many, many years, you're bound to think that it's part of the clinical picture, but here you'll see people who are alert, who clean windows, who do the dishes, clear the table, etc. You might think: these residents don't have dementia, they're too healthy for that. But that's not the case. It's the system that renders people apathetic.'

'That's a pretty bold statement,' I say.

'Yes, but it's true,' she replies confidently. 'If you want to provide good care you can't be afraid, so we go for nice walks in the woods here and we let people deliver the mail on site or weed the garden. We feed the animals together and everybody takes the stairs. Because they walk and move more, people are less likely to fall and if it does happen they're stronger.' Francien gives me one of her typical looks, as if to say: pretty obvious, right? 'Give residents the opportunity to strengthen their muscles in this way and they'll be both happier and more active for longer during this final stage of their life. And I'm not making this up, because Eindhoven University of Technology has done research here and their findings confirm it. I think it's also one of the reasons why residents here tend to live much longer than they do in a mainstream nursing home. There they last an average of six to eight months, while here it's two-and-a-half years. And the final phase, in which people are often confined to their beds, is much shorter here. If you prioritise quality of life, quantity will follow.'

'You make it all sound so logical.'

'Care is about people, and no two people are identical, and that includes those with dementia. Look at what works for them, what they like, and be kind to them. If you can do that, you can come and work here. You learn the practical side of things along the way. That's my logic. It's something that ordinary life has taught me, but it applies just as readily to care.

And about that care: we've gone straight into the deep end, and I haven't even offered you coffee yet. Let's have a cuppa.'

After coffee – with cream cake to celebrate our arrival – Francien and I walk around the yard where we bump into the farm's 'postman'. All the letterboxes have been affixed to a large wooden scaffold, which has the names of the residents on it in elegant lettering. After Thijs has taken the letters and parcels out of his trolley, he carefully slips them into the letterboxes, checking everything three times to ensure he doesn't make mistakes.

'Are you expecting a parcel today?' Thijs asks when he sees us watching.

'No, not today. But others do by the looks of it,' Francien replies.

'Absolutely. I'm very busy, so I'd better get on with it,' he says and picks up the next piece of mail.

Via the letterboxes we end up in the courtyard garden, where a member of staff and two residents are cuddling newborn puppies. Francien says: 'Every nursing home in the Netherlands should have something like this, whether it's kittens, guinea pigs, rabbits or dogs. What's better than looking after a bunch of cute little creatures together? It adds some structure to the day and encourages you to go outside, natural stimuli that lead to interaction, but more importantly, lots of moments of happiness. That's another thing ordinary life has taught me.'

Nearby, Ties is sitting under the chestnut tree, savouring his *Bolknak* cigar and the hustle and bustle in the garden, and a moment later we walk past Uncle Cor, who's drinking an ale under the overhang of his Hansel and Gretel cottage.

'It may all be "ordinary" to you,' I tell Francien, 'but that's not what it looks like to me. If so, it's the most ordinary paradise I've seen in my life. Even a lot of people without dementia would love to live here. I'm serious. The houses are all so charming, and everything has been made with so much love that it looks centuries old. Whether it's the wooden beams in my house, the classic gable end on Uncle Cor's cottage, the chic bistro chairs in the gardens, the beautiful flowerbeds with the hydrangeas and the elegant chestnut gates – nothing's been left to chance.'

'True, we've got Doris to thank for that. She travels the country to pick up "old junk" and overstock and works with the handymen to turn them into these treasures. She says that everything that's built here should have a lived-in feel, and as you can see, it creates an entirely different atmosphere than if we replaced the interiors every couple of years with items bought from medical or other specialist furniture companies. We want the informal carers, children, relatives and friends to like coming here and to have pleasant spaces where they can enjoy spending time together. I know this will sound really obvious again, but I can't repeat it often enough: it creates a richer and better life and doesn't cost a penny extra.'

'Is that right?' I ask. 'Because you do have a different financing structure.'

'That's correct,' Francien confirms. 'You can say what you like about the care sector in the Netherlands, but not that there's no scope for doing things differently. Anyone with dementia can choose their own care instead of outsourcing the decisions to a care administration office. They can use their personal budget and together with their informal carer put together a care package. We also receive some additional public funding, so we can often deliver this kind of care at the same price or even less. It means that everybody, regardless of income or savings, can live here, that's the beauty of it. An additional advantage is that we're not bound by nursing home legislation and therefore have greater freedom to shape the care we provide. I'm talking about the overall structure here, because of course we still get inspections.

I've noticed that all of us in the care sector are quick to find reasons why changes are impossible, and when things are done differently we look critically at whether or not it works. If we were more encouraging of those who are trying something new, I think we'd be moving faster in the right direction. I'm not saying this for our own benefit, because we've found our path, but for the many other organisations who'd like to do similar things but are afraid of being punished for mistakes along the way.' Francien shrugs her shoulders and gives me another one of those 'am I right' looks.

Just then, a care assistant comes out of the house and yells: 'Francien, there are people waiting for you outside Grootenhout I.'

'Totally slipped my mind. I'll be right there!' She turns to me. 'I'll come and find you later, okay?'

'Fine by me,' I say and walk back to 'my' house.

In the days that follow I realise just how much this vision penetrates every aspect of the organisation. For instance, my housemates and I are picked up by Taxi Sjarrel (the driver's name) for a cuppa at another farm. As part of these 'homecoming experiences', residents go out in the morning and afternoon to socialise at one of the other locations. It's fun and it breaks the daily routine, but even more importantly it lifts the residents' spirits.

'They may forget the actual experience, but the emotion

lingers,' is another one of Francien's one-liners that I totally agree with. Even something as simple as being collected in the taxi creates a special atmosphere and prompts lots of conversations in the car about things we see en route and about previous trips. It would never happen if you kept the residents inside all day, and it just goes to show: investing in people always pays off.

This is illustrated by another resident, Toos, who can usually be found in the kitchen. Her daughter told me that she came here in a wheelchair when she had literally nowhere else to go; nursing homes didn't know what to do with her. Toos talked nonstop all day, which other people found hard to deal with, and she was given more and more medication to stop that behaviour. But while it curbed the incessant talking, it also robbed her of her capacity to eat and walk unaided. Now that the medication has been reduced, Toos can once more communicate with her daughter, feed herself again and her mobility has improved to the extent that she no longer needs a wheelchair. The loquaciousness has come back too, so she often helps with jobs around the house or else the care assistants take her into the kitchen with them if it all becomes a bit too much for her fellow residents. Everything is done to stimulate rather than sedate Toos.

At first, many of these options appear to represent the more difficult path, because everything is more laborious, but the effort pays off in happier residents and relatives, as well as a more dynamic work environment for the carers. Besides, the fact that individual residents experience less fear, anger and sadness has a positive impact on the overall group, which in turn means less pressure at work. In short, it's a win-win situation.

While I'm having a coffee outside in the sun on my final day, I'm joined by Francien and Riek. 'You look like a cheeky monkey.' Riek says to me and laughs. She has the same lack of inhibition as Wil, but hers is expressed through language, a bit like Tourette's. But this disinhibition disappears as soon as she starts singing, and as a former opera singer she loves showing off her skills.

'Thank you, Riek, that's something I don't hear very often,' I say so as not to add fuel to the fire. Then she slumps in her seat and lets the sun do its job.

'Did you have a nice time?' Francien asks me.

'You've all created a very special place. I can genuinely say that I lived here for a few days, not merely survived, as is often the case in my nursing home. I've enjoyed my alert and quick-witted housemates, the gorgeous surroundings and the loving care in the various houses. And what struck me the most: at no point did I feel confined.'

'That's great to hear. Thank you,' says Francien, who's visibly touched. 'That's what we aim for here, and as for that final point, it's because we don't lock our doors. People can sense that. Keeping the doors unlocked is the best thing you can do. Our premise is: you're free to go, so you choose to stay. When you know the door is open, you feel much more relaxed, so much more at ease. As soon as someone locks that door and tells you "You're not allowed to leave until I say so," you no longer feel comfortable. You want to leave.'

'Doesn't anyone ever "escape", so to speak?'

'Absconding, running away, it hardly ever happens. And when it does, it's not a problem. We talk to the families about it in our intake interviews, and tell them that such risks are part of our ambition to provide a good life, and luckily they're fully behind that. It works quite well for most people;

they just like to know that they're free. And who can blame them? We've noticed that if we create a pleasant environment, they're less likely to leave and when they do go they come back quite quickly. Not that long ago, your housemate Ben suddenly got it into his head that he wanted to go to the supermarket round the corner from where he used to live. He simply had to get off the farm, so we let him and monitored the situation. He'd gone barely thirty-five metres before he returned because he wasn't very familiar with the "new neighbourhood" that had sprung up and wanted to come back home. It meant that we didn't have to go to extremes to calm Ben down. He was free to explore his feelings and then retreat to a safe space.

Being locked up scares people and makes them want to leave. Then they kick off and their so-called "problem behaviour" sets the whole medical machinery in motion. But it's our own fault: residents tell us they're scared and want to leave, but we tell them they're wrong to feel that way and maybe give them a pill to calm down. If we listened to what people with dementia are trying to tell us and we made the interior world more attractive than the one outside you'd be surprised how few people still want to leave.'

'Exactly,' I agree. 'Standing up for your vision from the word go, being clear about the risks and discussing them openly with the family and informal carers, scary as it may be, it all goes a long way. Let's face it, when freedom works well for the vast majority, we can't lock up all sick people as a group just because one or two might struggle a bit. To begin with, we must accept that life comes with risks and that none of these risks go away following a dementia diagnosis. Or as you would say: let's keep living "ordinary" lives.'

'Right you are!'

The dominant narrative

Amsterdam, the Netherlands

'What's dementia?' I ask.

'That's a very good question,' Anne-Mei says. Professor Anne-Mei The, who's in her fifties and dressed in powerful black, is a trained cultural anthropologist and holds the special chair in long-term care and dementia at VU Amsterdam University. She is also the founder of the Social Approach to Dementia, a movement that aims to give people with dementia a life that meets their needs and to help them strengthen and expand their social safety net.

'According to the dominant narrative in our society it's a terrible brain disease that encompasses a range of potentially very destabilising disorders. But after years of research, I've discovered a different story, which is rather more important: the story told by people with dementia themselves. They're telling us: "This disease is very unpleasant indeed, but the worst thing is that those around me no longer take me seriously, that they pity me, fall silent whenever I enter the room, exchange meaningful glances when I forget something, as if to say: oh, so that's how sick he is. Or: can we still trust what he says?" It's not that people with dementia experience gross discrimination, it's more subtle than that. Both in their private and professional lives, they're no longer seen as fully human or as the person they once were by those around them.

So the definition of dementia depends on who you're asking. Doctors will say something different from nurses or the people with dementia and their loved ones. And it's important to square all those different stories. We need to abandon that one dominant narrative about the brain and about loss and start telling the whole story.'

The place where Anne-Mei and I have spent the past few days, Huis van de Tijd (the House of Time), is part of this movement. Located in a beautiful old canal house in the centre of Amsterdam, it welcomes visitors with and without dementia and sets out to help people live at home for as long as possible. Anne-Mei and I are sitting at a round wooden table in one of the 'chill rooms' in the annex overlooking the courtyard. The light slanting through the high windows and onto the olive-green walls and matching sofa adds to the warm atmosphere.

It may be close to home, but this visit is another milestone. Anne-Mei was one of the first advisors to come on board, and now, two-and-a-half years and several countries later, we meet again.

'The Social Approach has really gathered momentum in recent years, hasn't it?' I remark. 'Have you seen a shift in the telling of this "other" story?'

'Yes, I think there's been a shift in the past eighteen months,' Anne-Mei says. 'Not least because what we say is now being corroborated by data, so the big players in the sector are starting to listen. But what's particularly important and meaningful to me is not that they're listening to me but to the people with dementia themselves. They're the ones who came up with this approach. What we want is for them to be heard.'

'In what sense did they come up with it? You're usually seen as the brains behind it.'

'True,' she says with a smile. 'Someone has to take the lead, as you know only too well. But that's not to say that it's my idea. We spent years following people with dementia from the first signs of cognitive decline until the end of their life. During the research, we always looked at what made them happy and we identified a pattern that explains where things go wrong. People with dementia are constantly asking for help in living their lives, and we respond to that request with care. That's the problem.

People with dementia are saying: "This illness doesn't just weigh on me as a patient, but it also has an impact on all the roles I've had in my life." It becomes harder for them to be a mother, father, brother, sister, lover. How can you help them continue in those capacities for as long as possible without ending up with unequal relationships? Their professional roles as carpenter, bank manager or engineer are compromised too. How can you prevent them from falling into a black hole when their diagnosis leaves them unfit for work, yet they still feel the need to be involved in their field and keep their mind agile? A final issue that people struggle with is their place in a social network or circle of friends. Whether it's a sports club, music society or other organisation, a neighbourhood or a school, they're all situations in which people's roles come under pressure. They often want help with that, but it's not forthcoming. It's as if, without meaning to, the minute someone is diagnosed we no longer see people for who they are and what they do, but just as patients. And as they tell us, that takes a bigger toll than the dementia itself.'

'It's weird,' I say. 'Many of the main problems that I've encountered in my nursing home and on our trip are staring us right in the face, and yet we're just not seeing them. People enter my home stripped of all their social roles, which is dehumanising and means that within weeks of becoming a "resident" they feel they no longer matter.'

'Exactly, it's dehumanising, and that's why it's so important to find out what our current approach to dementia is doing to people. Originally, dementia was a matter for doctors – "it's a brain disease" – and then came the psychologists who explained that it's a psychosocial problem too and tried to determine how best to deal with people with dementia. What we anthropologists do is we look at the bigger picture. Dementia is more than just an illness or an ill person. It includes the environment. Context matters. How we're seen by those around us matters, perhaps more than we ever imagined. That's why I love it that you're spending the day here with Rob and Joeri. I'm sure they'll show you things that I could never explain, not even in a thousand words.'

I check the time on my phone. 'Speaking of which: I promised to pick them up on my bike, so I'll catch you later, okay?'

'It's a deal,' Anne-Mei says.

Forty-five minutes later I press the golden doorbell of an elegant building in Amsterdam Oud-Zuid. A friendly voice over the intercom asks: 'Who is it?'

'Hi Rob, it's Teun. Are you coming? I've got Joeri beside me here.'

'Nice. I'll be down in two minutes.'

Besides Anne-Mei, Rob and Joeri are the main reason for our visit to the capital. Both men still live at home with their wives and children and go to the Huis van de Tijd a couple of days a week to spend some time together and talk to other people with dementia about what matters to them and how they can make these things happen.

Many of us think that we either won't get dementia or – if we do – only when we're old and on the scrapheap anyway, but alas, sometimes the reality is different. Dementia doesn't discriminate and can happen to us all regardless of age, gender and ethnicity. It doesn't care who or what you are. Both of the men I'm meeting today are younger than my father. Joeri (56), a tall, rugged guy with grey hair and bright blue eyes, was a creative in the advertising industry when he was diagnosed, while until recently Rob (54) was one of Europe's best cardiologists.

Early-onset dementia is relatively rare; according to the latest figures from the leading dementia organisations, some 15,000 people are afflicted in the Netherlands and around 3.9 million worldwide. But while uncommon, this form of the disease is often more aggressive. Due to the young age and faster progression, the changes have a particularly severe impact, because like these two men most people are still in the prime of their social and working life when diagnosed.

'Ah, there he is!' I exclaim when Rob walks through the door in his army-green jacket, jeans and brown suede shoes. He makes his way to his bike, which is parked beside a tree. Rob is about the same height as Joeri and has similar blue eyes but a less abundant head of hair.

'I think we'll have to pedal fast to avoid a soaking, so let's go,' Joeri says, whereupon the two men hop on their bikes.

I have to push hard to keep up with them. Normally, Rob and Joeri ride together, but because I'm keen to see what an independent life with dementia looks like, I'm joining them today on this route through Amsterdam.

'So cycling and navigating isn't a problem for you?' I ask when we stop at a traffic light.

'Not a problem at all,' Joeri says. 'So we'll carry on as long as we can...'

'Exactly,' Rob says. 'We'll keep doing our thing.'

The light turns green, and we ride via Frederiksplein towards Magere Brug. The light-hearted nature of our conversation is familiar to me, as my housemates tend to use to it conceal what's really going on. So I'm curious to find out how these two tough guys are handling the drastic changes and their grim life expectancy.

When we get to the long table in the living room of the House of Time and drape our coats over the backs of the chairs, I notice Joeri's shiny Rolex. 'Nice piece of bling,' I say.

'Yes, I still love beautiful things.' He smiles.

Seeing this ultimate status symbol of success, I'm even more interested to know how they experience their life now that they're no longer part of the corporate jungle. 'What was it like, Joeri, when you'd always been creative, when you'd made it your profession, to realise that it was all about to change?'

'It was a hard pill to swallow,' Joeri says. 'I denied it for a long time, for at least one or two...' There's a silence as he searches for the right word. 'Hey, I can't think of the word,' he says in frustration.

'Years?' I suggest tentatively.

'Yes, that's what I meant.'

'And how did your partner respond?'

'My wife stopped laughing at my jokes,' Joeri says with a bit of a chuckle.

'Ah, that's a bummer,' I reply in the same breezy tone. 'And may I ask what form of dementia you have?'

There's another brief silence, and Joeri shifts restlessly in his seat. 'Where's the card that says what it is?' he wonders, rifling through his coat pockets.

'Fronto-temporal dementia? Lewy body dementia?' I prompt him.

'Yes, Lewy body, that's it.' He takes a relieved breath.

Lewy body is a form of dementia caused by clumps of protein in the brain, deposits known as Lewy bodies. It can lead to all kinds of symptoms, including problems with thinking, movement and behaviour.

'Do you suffer from hallucinations?' I ask. 'Because that's common with this variant, isn't it?'

'It comes and goes. Not at the moment, but sometimes it gets so bad it's impossible to ignore. For instance, I once spent a lot of time with a gnome. I could actually see it and talk to it. My wife used to say: "Darling, there is no gnome, honestly..." That's tough, I can tell you.' Joeri heaves a deep sigh. 'It's like I'm on a gentle slide, and without even realising it I just keep sliding further down. It's pretty scary. During hallucinations, I often feel as if I'm screaming for help and nobody hears me. And what's even scarier is knowing that while I still have some control over the hallucinations now, that too will go. I feel as if I'm being slowly taken over by something that's destroying every last bit of Joeri and that will keep going until there's nothing left.'

I look at him, devastated. The reality of what it must be like to live with this prospect hits me harder than ever before, and his fear and uncertainty about what's to come seem to fill the room.

'That's why I'm so happy here,' he says after a long silence.

'Really, how come?'

'In here it's not weird when I talk about things like that, because people understand. That's certainly not a given. Look, I obviously didn't talk to my colleagues about gnomes,' he jokes, 'but the looks I get from acquaintances when we chat or I pass them in the street can really hurt. It's as if I'm no longer in any way, shape or form connected to the man they once liked. You turn into a second-rate citizen overnight whereas you actually need a helping hand when you're going through all these difficult and scary things. I've been living with this for a few years now and it's the one thing that's remained the same. It needs to change.'

'Is that what you think as well, Rob?' I ask.

'You bet,' says Rob, who's been all ears. 'As a cardiologist I used to fly around the globe to speak at prestigious conferences, but since my diagnosis I've neither seen hide nor hair of my colleagues, not a soul. If anyone ought to understand what's happening to me it's them. But as Joeri says: no matter how important you were, for many people you literally cease to exist after you're diagnosed.'

Just then a door opens and an older lady in an arty purple jogging suit exclaims: 'Gentlemen, it's time for a glass and a dance. How about it?'

'Wonderful, Brigitte!' the two friends respond almost in unison.

'Do you know what it is, Teun?' Joeri says as he stands up. 'We just want to live and enjoy what little time we have left. We have to deal with the situation, whether we like it or not. But everything around it can be changed, so it's time for a revolution. And I've got a few ideas about the design.' He laughs and gives me a mischievous look. 'Come, let's liven this place up. Any requests?

At that, Rob jumps up as well and says: 'Dire Straits, always good!'

When the wine is served and the music blasts through the building, more visitors start trickling in and the somewhat sober living room transforms into a red-hot dance venue. Everybody starts shaking their hips like nobody's watching. When Anne-Mei is the last one to walk through the door she's encouraged to hit the dance floor amidst much cheering. She doesn't need to be told twice.

After a few songs I join Anne-Mei on the steps outside the building for a chat while the festivities continue indoors. 'Rob and Joeri's stories left me speechless,' I say. 'I can see that they dread the prospect of moving into a nursing home, where they'll have to share their living room with a waltzing violin player on telly. Their lives were so different before they were diagnosed, and you can tell that they're afraid of losing their social roles altogether. Does the care sector really need a paid service, like the Social Approach, that teaches us to be more sociable and mitigate this? Can't we just treat each other differently?'

'I wish,' Anne-Mei replies. 'Unfortunately, it doesn't work that way in practice. It really takes a radical shake-up for us as a society to change our attitude to people with dementia. It's not something we can decide between ourselves. For a structural change you need to get the masses on board, and they need help, which requires money, unfortunately.

To start with, you need coaches to help organisations and local councils understand why we need a different perspective. Next up, you need teams that oversee the implementation of these changes over a period of time so there's a degree of acceptance in the organisation and the vision becomes embedded in everyday practice. Change takes time, and you need to give people space and not put them off with a transition that's too sudden or too extreme. Because let's be honest, it's quite a shock to no longer be judged on whether the floor is clean, dinner is served at the correct temperature or nobody has fallen, but on how happy your residents are. Social activities must come to be seen as vital components of happiness, to help people understand what effect they have and why they're so important. Did Mr Steggerda enjoy his outing to the supermarket? Did Jannie have a nice chat and did Mark get the chance to play his favourite music to his housemates?

It may sound a bit childish to name these things, to make them an explicit part of the system, but once we're used to working in this way it will mark the beginning of a step change. People like to have some control over the job they do, so giving them a framework is one way of building the necessary confidence.'

'But how does that work in practice for people like Rob and Joeri?'

'The most important thing to us here is to empower people, to coach them, to make use of the skills they never lose and thus restore as much self-confidence as possible. From the moment our visitors arrive here, they really come back into their own, which has a hugely positive impact on their home situation.

At the same time we try to reorganise the social network around them. The men probably told you that after a while those communities totally disintegrate. We try to address that as a team by having talks with the various social groups in the life of the dementia sufferer and see how those people can contribute to a more meaningful existence. And we're not seeing any reluctance or lack of understanding on those individuals' parts. Quite the opposite: they're only too happy to become involved. They tell us that they felt paralysed by the diagnosis. What should I do, they wondered. Is there anything I can do? Does my friend or colleague still need me? So in the end the distance between them increases and the safety net disappears. We're trying to achieve the exact opposite with our approach, so people no longer die a social death after they're diagnosed, but actually strengthen their social network.

What we're doing here builds on the support we give at home. We help the people who come here to choose how they want to spend their days and evenings, so it's not the dementia that takes centre stage, but their needs as a human being. It boosts their quality of life, which is so important to them in this phase. Because we help people design their own safety net, both here and at home, they can keep going and keep doing the things that matter to them for longer while also feeling stronger and more human. And ultimately, they can live at home for longer, which is what many of them really want.'

'I agree, it's admirable to listen more to what people themselves need,' I say. 'Nobody wants to leave their home, but wouldn't you say that people often cling to this notion of living at home when it's just not possible anymore? I get the impression that a nursing home is often the last resort when the informal carer is literally at breaking point.'

'Yes, exactly. That's what makes the situation so depressing,' Anne-Mei says. 'I've seen so many cases of informal carers who interpreted the deterioration of their partner as a personal failure, ended up trying even harder and sometimes literally buried themselves in caring for their loved one. In fact, three-quarters of informal carers die earlier than their peers and sometimes even before the person with dementia they were looking after. That's incredibly sad. By creating a safety net for the person with dementia at an early stage we're automatically doing the same for the caregiver, so we're relieving some of the burden and helping them care for longer. We ought to interpret "coexistence" in the broadest sense of the word: not just as two or more people living together in a house, but as living with everybody around you, in a community. We have to have the courage to invest in that, with clear financing in place, so informal carers don't get crushed by their work, but actually receive the help they need.

It's not a question of simply pouring in more money, but of investing differently. That also calls for a different approach from the government, which has to come up with new criteria for how the money is invested. I hope that in the years to come we'll see plenty more social initiatives that will help with this, so that ultimately all needs are catered for, and coexistence becomes the norm. When that happens we will have effectively worked ourselves out of a job as initiators. That's the goal!'

'Are you guys still sitting there?' asks Joeri from the hallway, and he comes and stands behind us. 'The party seems to be winding down, but Rob and I were thinking of having one for the road at Brasserie Van Dam, which is just round the corner from Rob's house. We're heading that way anyway...' He gives us another one of his mischievous looks.

'You know me so well, Joeri,' Anne-Mei says. 'But I'm already late for my next appointment. But I think Teun and Jonathan are up for a beer. What do you say, guys?'

'You bet, more than one in fact,' I react.

Joeri turns round and yells down the hallway: 'Rob, I've talked them into it. Let's head off...'

XI A new horizon

A global conclusion

Norway – Switzerland – the Netherlands – Slovenia – Moldova – the United States – Belgium – South Korea – Denmark – Sweden – South Africa

Why does change happen so incredibly slowly when most of the people I speak to would do things differently tomorrow if they could? It's a question that preoccupies me throughout our trip. Of course, I know I'm not the first to wonder about this and I certainly won't be the last. With each country I visit and each person I meet, my impression grows that change is something we all long for but struggle to initiate. I feel that as soon as action is called for, we look to others to take responsibility. We think something is too big for us to tackle on our own, too small to make an immediate impact, too complicated to do, or else we're scared of being a trailblazer or think it's no longer cool when too many people are calling for something.

But the great thing about change is that it's a process that never stops. And that process really ought to take the form of a question, as described so eloquently by Carla Molenberghs, the founder of that lovely nursing home in Belgium, the one that used all those warm materials: 'Every change must be rooted in a vision that aims for an ideal, and most importantly that vision must always remain a topic of conversation. That's why it ought to be formulated as a series of questions: is this right? Do I agree? What do others think? In this way, you're always collectively working on happiness, and on a constantly changing world that will endure.'

I can't stop thinking about this line of reasoning and the more I think about it the more I suspect that this striving towards an ideal may also be the greatest obstacle to real change.

Striving for something so big can lead to many disappointments along the way, and with the end goal feeling overly idealistic or impossible many people may be quick to give up. This often means that as well as the ideal itself, any good things that have been achieved in the process end up dead and buried too. So we need a different approach. As Francien van de Ven, the manager of the care farm in Brabant, puts it: 'We must give more encouragement to those who are trying to change, and create a culture in which the courage to change trumps the fear of failure.'

It all begins with setting achievable goals, however small they may be. At the same time, we must celebrate and share every little success, because success will sell any message, especially one of hope. As Jonathan said when we were exploring how we might tell the story of dementia in a different way: 'We should take a leaf out of Coca-Cola's book. Success isn't a goal, but a means to tell your story. If we believe that we've already achieved success and all we need to do is share it, we can never fail.'

The beauty of it is that after everything I've seen around the world, I know how much we've already won and I don't just *believe* that this hopeful future is possible, I *know* it. We just need to share examples of this success, or as the people behind the well-known soft drink would say: 'Share the happiness.'

Happiness in mainstream care

Like large-scale mainstream care, small-scale private care has to contend with a major preconception. Everything is supposed to be easier because there are fewer residents, the homes are better and more modern and the atmosphere homelier. While that's true of many of the smaller care homes I've seen, it doesn't necessarily lead to happy residents.

In other words: form never eclipses function. However beautiful the homes I see may be, real happiness always originates in a vision. My experience at a large nursing home in Belgium is a great illustration of this. The minute I entered, I wanted to turn around and leave again. Another one of those sad places, I thought to myself. But that feeling melted away as soon as I realised that people were treated with more loving care than I'd ever seen in a home of this size. 'The best medicine for people with dementia is physical proximity,' I'm told by Patricia Bauters, ward manager at Aymonshof nursing home. 'If there's always a care assistant close by, nobody need ever be distressed. I teach the carers here to treat the residents like their own mother or father. And whether it's domestic staff or management, we all look after one another. It changes everything.'

This becomes clear when a woman is seen tugging at the closed door. She seems a little angry and fearful. A carer who's serving coffee walks straight over to her and says: 'Hey Feline, what is it? What's bothering you? I'm so sorry, is there anything I can do to help?' Then she gives the woman a big hug. This quick response is admirable in and of itself, and the mode of address even more so, but what happens next goes any further. While gently rubbing Feline's back, the care worker takes her to her room, where she puts on the woman's favourite French music and lies down next to her on the bed. The result is instant calm, and as soon as Feline has nodded off, the carer goes back to the coffee.

There's no arguing with residents over where their home is, which only exacerbates the situation, and no pill in their apple sauce to avoid such scenes. Just a different outlook, which in turn leads to a different outcome. 'Getting to know somebody and finding out what his or her needs are and then acting accordingly – while allowing and acknowledging any emotions there may be – we believe that's the only correct way of dealing with people with dementia,' Patricia tells me when she sees how moved I am. 'They live in an eternal present. Their past is fading and the future doesn't mean much to them, so that's why we must respect their 'now' as much as we can.

What we're seeing at this nursing home in Dendermonde is that all the beautiful objects, materials and innovations in the world can never create the loving approach prompted by this simple yet brilliant vision. That's not to say that all other efforts are irrelevant – far from it, they can make the care system even better. What it boils down to is that a home begins with loving contact on the ground and not with trendy terms such as 'person-centred care' and 'autonomy' on websites. And it doesn't matter how big or small a nursing home is; this vision and approach can have an impact anywhere. This is in no way diminished by the fact that this home still has some way to go when it comes to unlocking doors, creating a cosier atmosphere and improving the quality of its food. On the contrary, if these are its biggest problems, then the future at Aymonshof looks very bright indeed.

My optimism about large-scale care is borne out by a visit to a nursing home on the Norwegian fjords, which is also seeking to improve the quality of life for people with a form of dementia. Again, I discover that real change doesn't begin with new regulations but with a cultural shift.

Upon arrival, all the usual stereotypes seem to be reinforced, but after a few minutes I sense that there's something remarkable going on. The care assistants are dressed in traditional uniforms and the décor is that of a typical nursing home divided into several 'houses', yet the residents look vibrant and happy. Like we've seen in other locations, the food is freshly cooked and there's music, but the real surprise here is a vision I've not encountered elsewhere: in an effort to boost happiness and interaction residents aren't allocated rooms on the basis of their diagnosis or indication, but on the basis of needs instead. What do they ask for? Who would they like to be with, and who not? Would they rather live upstairs or downstairs, adjacent to the garden or close to the living room? But the main difference with the other homes is that the houses are made completely stimulus-free for those who are highly sensitive to stimuli.

Most of the people in these houses have frontotemporal dementia, a form that many believe requires extra attention because it can lead to impulsive behaviour. It's a huge challenge for carers. In Germany, for example, we visited a home that accommodates residents with this form of dementia from all over the country, because many nursing homes struggle to provide the right kind of care. To avoid the overstimulation that often leads to impulsive behaviour, the living room in Norway looks as if everybody has only just moved in and the removal van with furniture has yet to arrive. Window film makes it all but impossible to look outside, and there are just enough chairs for the residents, plus one extra. When they're in this room the residents receive one-on-one attention, because the staff found that it makes them less fearful and aggressive. Sometimes they even begin to display atypical, positive behaviour and end up seeking out stimuli and their fellow residents again. It goes to show that we shouldn't always start from our own perspective, because however bleak this kind of bare environment may feel to an outsider, it can be effective for the people that live here and need it.

This approach transformed the dynamic at the nursing home practically overnight and now there's little or no agitation. The outcome is astonishing: active, happy people who spend the day together in the garden or in one of the living rooms, so the other houses can manage with just a single care assistant and antipsychotics have only been used once in the past five years.

From the outside this looks like typical nursing home care, but an enlightened vision makes the inside feel like a home of the future. There is no culture of fear here; nobody is scared of making mistakes or of being blamed for something, as I see elsewhere. The type of care offered is always open for discussion, and a lot of thought goes into providing care that really benefits the residents. Happiness is not measured by a strict checklist, but by the degree of activity and interaction among residents, including those who can no longer walk unaided. The staff try to get inside residents' heads by listening to them instead of having 'them' listen to 'us'. The default response to incidents is not to lock doors or increase medication. On the contrary. A team meeting is called to see what the organisation and the staff can do differently to prevent something similar from happening in the future. The resulting openness and support proves that the necessary change in large-scale nursing home care is not light years away, but just around the corner.

I saw a similarly enlightened approach to care in Slovenia. Within a relatively short time, a group of scholars led by Professor Zvezdan Pirtošek has managed to put care for people with dementia on the map in the southern European nation. Because family ties are more important here than in many Western countries, there was some debate initially as to which corner of the world might serve as a role model, but ultimately they decided to forge their own path. It resulted in a number of progressive insights, the most eye-catching of which is the 'positive care incentive'.

When we visited a nursing home about a ten-minute drive from Ljubljana, we were told that instead of being given extra cash for more seriously ill patients the organisation is rewarded for healthier people. It removes the perverse care incentive that's the norm in the Netherlands, where institutions are all trying to attract people with a more complex care indication to obtain more money. The positive care incentive means that this Slovenian nursing home is now doing all it can to keep people fit. Not only are the residents enjoying exercise sessions, but social clubs are popping up all over the grounds, which creates the impression of being in a small village rather than a nursing home. The upshot is that the residents are both healthier and happier.

Not long after, we arrive in Balstahl, a small Swiss border town, where I witness one of the most traditional health care systems I've ever seen. The moment we set foot inside and the roles of the various care assistants are explained to us, the hierarchy is evident. But it also shows how more money can lead to more problems in a care system. Doctors here earn commission on the medication they prescribe, so most of the people in this expensive, state-of-the-art building are completely apathetic. Luckily, I also speak with a brave care manager who's standing up to this and is slowly making headway in this traditional and hierarchical system – not by antagonising anyone, but by coming up with real-life illustrations that show that the residents are people, first and foremost. Instead of being silenced, they should be allowed to find their own equilibrium in the later stages of life. According to the manager in question, Gina Kunst, the greatest challenge is that the quality of care in Switzerland is assessed on 'paper' care rather than 'actual' care. This has also been one of my biggest bugbears in my own country.

One of the main excuses for not changing is that daily admin is simply taking too much time. People would be seriously outraged if they saw the size of my housemates' electronic client dossiers (ECDs) and the time spent on this paperwork by those who ought to make a difference on the ground. Nobody seems to wonder where these checklists came from and whether we should continue to use them. I understand that this may be difficult for some, but please ask yourself: why? Who benefits from registering the colour, smell and shape of every stool?

The resident? No.

The care assistant? No.

The management? No.

The inspectors? No.

The family? No.

The legal guardian? No.

The doctor or geriatrician? Maybe?

I'm simplifying matters to get my point across, but do we really need to track this kind of information for everyone? Or should the need for such a medical report be decided on a case-by-case basis? We know that the nursing home is the terminus for those that live there, so shouldn't we be asking ourselves if and how the data contribute to any happiness experienced at this stage in life? Because sadly this is just one of many things that the organisation wants to see logged or reported. It's as if we've drawn up a set of rules so we don't have to think for ourselves and certainly don't have to accept responsibility. A while back, I overheard some care assistants discussing an incident registration (via a so-called MIC, or *melding incident client* in Dutch) they had to fill in, and it captured the problem more eloquently than I ever could.

'How is it possible that Mrs Van Ginkel fell a second time this week?'

'No idea. I just checked, but her file didn't mention anything unusual.'

'Hmm, I see...'

Let's chuck out all these files, reports and checklists and give carers the space to look, talk, feel and listen. Let's remember that people spend the final stage of their life in a nursing home and would like individual attention, not a print-out of their stay. I genuinely believe that this is the way to attract more staff (and not just medically trained personnel), which is one of the most pressing challenges facing the care sector at the moment. With less box ticking, carers can start to give more attention to residents. The number of managers can also be halved, as less monitoring equals less managing and more space for actual rather than paper care.

I witnessed a step in the right direction recently when I

gave a talk to an organisation where everybody, director and management included, was expected to work as a carer one day a week. After a great deal of initial resistance, it was soon warmly embraced by all involved. The measure not only led to mutual understanding on many levels, but it also structurally increased carer numbers without the need to employ more staff. A good example of effective management, if you ask me.

Another issue that could improve quality of life – one of the most talked about issues in recent years and something I've long campaigned for – is the end to locked doors. In the places I've visited that didn't have their doors locked, the impact on resident happiness was off the scale. Weirdly, almost everybody thinks that residents will abscond in droves as soon as the door opens, but the opposite is true. It's the sense of being trapped that makes people more fearful and therefore more inclined to want to leave. Again, there's cause for optimism as more and more people and organisations are starting to change this. One such person is the manager of Huize Hunderen in the Dutch village of Twello. Care innovator Michiel van Putten tells me:

> 'Why does everything have to be safe? Unlock the doors! We've made things very difficult for ourselves in the healthcare sector. Everything is about risk aversion and making sure that money is being spent wisely. That alone creates a mountain of paperwork, and it gets even worse when the inspectors come round and we all freak out when we're asked: "How do you keep people safe?" Why not think: let's consult with the family and give everybody as much freedom as possible and the best quality of life. But no, what

happens is we draw up endless checklists, so we have a log of everything we do. And that's where the trouble starts. I try to fight it by asking the staff: why does it have to be safe? Life is full of risk, so why should it be any different now? Over the past four decades in the Netherlands, we've become quite good at watching every penny, and then on top of it all we try to quantify people's quality of life. We need to accept that freedom involves risks. Whether or not they have dementia, people in their seventies and eighties are more prone to falling, and that's partly because their sense of balance is not as good as it used to be. But is that a reason to stick them in a chair all day? That's so unhealthy! Let's make the transition from shelters where people are kept safely alive to vibrant homes where people get on with their lives, however risky that may be.'

People like Michiel give me hope, because they show us that there's a different way and by doing so remove the fear of the unknown in those who are scared that their loved one will walk off as soon as the doors are opened. And what if that happens? How bad would it be after months or even years of confinement? These questions invariably point me in the direction of solutions that seem straightforward, but that are still exceptions to the rule.

Turn nursing homes into places where we would want to live. Don't update the interior every five years with identikit furnishings but create a cosy atmosphere like May does in Denmark, Carla in Belgium and Francien in the Netherlands. A place where real things, real plants and real animals combine to make a pleasant environment, and where the food is fresh and tasty, because that too still matters in the final stages of life. So don't encourage residents to drink tea and coffee all day long, and don't just serve white sliced bread for breakfast and lunch, followed by bland, mushy food for dinner. Accept that people are still active participants in life and don't need to be 'fed' three times a day.

Make nursing homes part of the community in which they're located, and don't just let the residents stare out of the window. Go outside and let the outside world in. Differentiate between the days of the week, and invite social neighbourhood initiatives, organisations and businesses to have their meetings or card games at the home once or twice a month. Involve residents in local schools, as is done in the US, without differentiating between the healthy and less healthy. Create lasting relationships and not one-off initiatives that are just for show. Let volunteers decide when to drop by; someone will always be up for a chat, a cuppa or a walk. Make sure they don't have to rearrange work and family commitments to visit, because then they may not keep coming. I, for one, have never felt galvanised by routine. Spontaneity, on the other hand, makes me feel alive.

Cherish differences, for instance by not grouping people with the same diagnosis together. Allow people of different ages and with different care needs to live side by side, as they do in Moldova. Form households in which daily activities create a bond, vibrancy and a meaningful structure to the day. Organise outings, however modest, like they do at the Grootenhout estate, which result in happy emotions that linger even if the activity itself is forgotten. Whether it's a cuppa on another unit, a stroll around the courtyard garden or a trip to the local bakery, anything goes as long as it's genuinely meaningful. And do your work with a smile – it's a superpower we all have and one that doesn't cost a thing, brings a lot of happiness and makes the world we work in so much nicer.

The beauty of such outings is that anyone can supervise them, so it's key that these activities are normalised, not medicalised. That way people without medical training can accompany the residents, giving the other care assistants more time to do their work.

Government-backed happiness

People who want to see changes in care often look to the government, expecting a group of omniscient officials to deliver happiness. While I don't believe they can, I've also seen the vacuum that's created when a country's leadership doesn't do anything to improve care for vulnerable people. What we certainly don't need is a government that lurches from term to term, handing out taxpayers' money to those groups that shout the loudest. I believe in an administration that has a vision and that takes it upon itself to break the stigma around dementia and improve the way the illness is seen. A vision isn't just the beating heart of good care, it must also guide those that look after our interests as a society.

It's essential that all people are treated equally under that vision. A government that keeps anyone segregated, in whatever way, creates exclusion. In that sense, the world's best-known care facility, the Dutch Hogeweyk dementia village, takes on an entirely new meaning for Rayne Stroebel, the prominent South African scholar from Hout Bay: 'Hogeweyk is nothing less than a ghetto for those with dementia. A place with walls to shield people from the outside world is by definition not inclusive, and this will always have a detrimental effect on happiness.' It's something I saw for myself when I found one of the residents there rattling the locked door. I would urge any government to invest in a vision that contributes to people's happiness by making sure they remain involved in society; by not being fixated on incidents, overstating their impact and using them as an excuse to propose rules for an entire group, but by always putting quality of life at the centre of the debate.

Then there are the organisations that claim to be acting in the best interests of people with dementia yet seem to be doing the opposite. How can we steer them in the right direction? The bulk of my fellow countrymen and women have a very distorted view of the secure unit where I've been living for three years, which is no surprise really, given all the terrifying TV programmes in which relatively young folk with dementia burst into tears because they can't remember their children's names and adverts with slogans such as 'Forget me not' and 'United against dementia'. Of course dementia can be frightening, difficult and painful for all those who are having to deal with it, but in the end these campaigns, however well-intentioned they may be, paint a very limited picture and could be doing more harm than good. The only answer that all these scaremongering campaigns come up with is money, and their appeals for donations yield millions and millions every year. It creates a cycle of fear with which the various interest groups and organisations consolidate their existence at the expense of the people they represent. It seems to have led to a system in which money is no longer a means but an end in itself.

A side effect of the focus on fundraising is that these scare campaigns tend to depict people with dementia in such a hopeless way that it doesn't seem to matter what happens to them because they're not compos mentis anyway. It's why my positive experiences at the nursing home often evoke reactions such as: 'Do they really have dementia, the people you live with?', 'Oh, in your place "they" are still "all there",' or 'I thought those people couldn't remember anything, let alone form friendships?'

When even the groups and organisations that look after the interests of those with dementia get their representation so wrong, then how can we expect a more open-minded and positive attitude from 'ordinary people'? The millions who have to live with some form of dementia today or tomorrow certainly don't benefit from 'their' advocates deepening the stigma as part of campaigns. If anything, it adds to the daily burden of loss and shame.

Of course, some of these charity millions go towards funding projects that improve the lives of people with dementia. But what good does that do when any positive changes are undone by the next campaign?

When it comes to dementia, most of the money is earmarked for research into the 'remedy' that will fix everything. Millions, billions even, are spent every year in the search for 'the miracle pill', but is that a fair distribution of funds when it remains to be seen whether a cure-all will ever be possible? As Professor Peter Whitehouse puts it: It's a myth to think that there will ever be that one pill, as most of the evidence now suggests that there isn't a single cause of dementia or Alzheimer's. So how many miracle cures will we need?

I think the search for more effective treatments is important, but I believe we can do more for more people if some of the millions are spent on the wellbeing of those who are living with dementia now and in the near future. So let's not focus too narrowly on 'curing', but keep striving for a healthier balance between the search for a cure and efforts to improve the quality of life. At the same time it's important to tell the whole story about people living with dementia around the world, and to be truthful about every single aspect, because of course dementia remains a destabilising condition that none of us want to live with. I'm not alone in wanting to grow old without any aches and pains and then, one sunny day, pass away peacefully under a tree. But the reality is usually different.

The government should also invest more in another approach that can greatly enhance quality of life: prevention. This will render the search for a miracle pill less relevant, because here too the time-honoured principle applies that prevention is better than cure. If people like nothing better than to age well and without a care in the world then why don't we focus all our efforts on this? Especially now that research from Sweden and South Korea has shown that there's a very real chance of preventing or delaying the onset of certain forms of dementia. These studies also show that prevention will always be more cost-effective, and pressure on the care sector will obviously fall sharply as patient numbers drop.

Help people live healthier lives by making healthy products cheaper and unhealthy foods pricier. Why are hamburgers still available for little over a euro, whereas you'd be hard-pressed to find a healthy equivalent for the same money? Make supermarkets as well as school and sports canteens something more than the glorified sugar factories they are now. Again, we should be even-handed. A glass of coke isn't going to give you diabetes tomorrow, but what if you drink it daily or weekly and also eat other unhealthy products? What does it do to your body? Why do we treat our health in this way when we're aware of the long-term consequences of our consumption habits, and diabetes and obesity figures are sky-rocketing? I urge any government to invest in healthier lifestyles by making wholesome food affordable to all, encouraging exercise and social interaction and stimulating lifelong learning. Learning new things creates new connections in the brain. You could compare it to building a network of motorways through your head: the more roads there are, the more ways you have of reaching your destination. If there are only a few routes, it doesn't take much for everything to become congested. So make sure to create as many thoroughfares as possible.

A final priority for the government should be the introduction of a transparent payment scheme, so that informal carers aren't sent from pillar to post when they're trying to access support. We won't see many more new nursing home places opening up in the future, and as a society we're going to have to deal with that. The state should help with this. Enable people to live at home for longer if that's what they want, but make sure that informal carers don't miss out because they have no idea how to apply for assistance. Give them the financial leeway to spend as much time as possible with their loved one during this very difficult period – and the best possible time too, so that like Arlene in South Africa they feel fortunate rather than hard done by.

Don't abandon people with dementia but look at how various initiatives and approaches might help them carry on as normal for as long as they can. Again, a new narrative is crucial, one that eases the fear of dementia so that people don't die a social death but are looked after by their network. Families, employers, clubs and neighbourhoods should all be encouraged to do this and be informed about the ways of making this happen, because as Joeri and Rob from Amsterdam taught us, the toughest thing for people with dementia may well be the reactions of those around them. This is how Anne-Mei put it to me: 'It's time to give dementia a bigger stage and to start listening to what people themselves have to say and how they see dementia. That way, we'll start to understand the importance of context in how we tell a story.'

Happiness is in the little things

The most important lesson I've learnt in three years of travelling around four continents and eleven countries is that the happiness we so crave is right under our noses. We have to learn to live together again. As Lia in Apeldoorn explained, a good quality of life begins with feeling that you matter, that you are of value. It's a universally powerful and relevant desire that cuts across nations and cultures, and that we can fulfil today by building communities that give people with dementia a sense of meaning and legitimacy. All those I met on my travels who felt excluded from society said they'd rather be dead than alive, whereas the opposite was true for those who felt seen by family, friends and neighbours. This leads me to believe that the biggest change of all will be within reach the moment we start telling different stories. Or as Professor Peter Whitehouse says: 'If we can just shift people's attitudes and say, "The real answer here is friendlier communities," then friendlier communities will help us all in the future. We will create happier lives for all of us, not just people with dementia.'

To achieve this, we need to change the dementia narrative and start telling a different story. We have to paint a more truthful picture of dementia and move from a world in which we want to manage the lives of people living with the condition to one in which we listen to how they want to live and then try to facilitate this for as long as possible. That's the difference between taking care of someone and genuinely caring for them. Instead of talking about people with dementia and responding to their needs with off-the-peg solutions, we ought to listen to them and help them with what they want. Until their very last breath.

Enable people to live at home for as long as possible by asking how this may be done, without the informal carer breaking down. It's up to us to help, and to the government to provide the funding as well as clear instructions on how to apply for it. Too often I hear from people that they don't know which pot of money pays for what, and I once acquired a new housemate because his partner and carer no longer knew how to finance everything at home. Surely this should never be a reason for moving into a nursing home?

Employers, trade unions and health and safety officials should team up with the government and see to it that people with dementia aren't immediately signed off work following a diagnosis but kept in employment for as long as possible. This may be done by offering them a shorter work week to make the job more manageable, exploring the option of a demotion after some time to reduce work pressure and focusing on the things they can still do.

In the same vein, sports clubs should try to retain people and neighbours should look out for one another. We can only deal with what's to come by working together. So don't abandon people with dementia, include them.

We must stop patting ourselves on the back by claiming that the Netherlands has the best healthcare in the world, when many of the people in our 18 billion euro system would rather be dead than alive. Surely that doesn't merit the qualifier 'best'? Let's change that narrative, too, by actually trying to achieve the best care in the world instead of being complacent and clinging to an illusion.

We ought to get rid of the idea that a nursing home is a

sanctuary for elderly people where nothing is allowed to happen. It has to be a *home*, one where normal life carries on where possible, and where you can hurt or burn yourself, choke on something or fall. Large-scale mainstream care could be amazing if we were to structure it differently, but for that you need those in charge to provide assurance that other approaches or more risks are acceptable and you won't be held accountable if something happens. Before committing someone to a home, children, friends and family, partners and informal carers have to have a conversation about where they're taking their loved one, what life there will be like, what the pros and cons are and who accepts responsibility.

Until we see people with dementia in a new light and create new frameworks for dealing with them, each new vision will fail. Person-centred care, autonomy – the websites make it look wonderful, but none of it means anything when safety and control remain paramount.

So let's create a framework in which trust rather than safety takes precedence, in which we trust care assistants to offer a form of care that's all about quality not quantity of life. This means that the day's activities can vary depending on a resident's individual needs or on those of the group as a whole, as long as everything starts from a sense of belonging and feeling as though you matter.

Early one morning, as I'm lying in bed in my room in Amstelveen, staring at the modular ceiling, I feel the spring sunshine touch my face through the net curtains. At that moment I realise that I've been living at this nursing home for three years. For three years I've seen the bright green leaves appear on the trees in the enclosed courtyard and for three years I've been dreaming that next spring will be different... I'm dreaming of a spring in which we're no longer behind closed doors and tall fences, but free to enjoy this time of year when everything looks just that little bit more hopeful and beautiful than before. And this spring that feeling of hope is stronger than ever. Why?

It's because I've spent the past three years looking at what a better quality of life might look like for people who are living with a form of dementia, now or in the future, and what I found surpassed my expectations. I encountered people, scientists and organisations that show that a different outlook definitely leads to a different outcome. I've seen many fine and loving examples of care, but above all I found a common denominator that's essential for a happier life and that's at the heart of what makes a good life: the feeling that you are of value, that you matter. And the great thing about this feeling is that it transcends all borders and all cultures and can therefore serve as a universal foundation, not just for a new method of care, but above all for a new way of living together. Good care isn't an individual achievement, it's the outcome of a collective effort.

A cry from the heart, part 2

My name is Teun Toebes,
and I still believe that people living with a form of dementia
aren't getting the attention they deserve.
That makes me incredibly sad.

But...

I'm hopeful – hopeful that we can create
a better and more inclusive future for people with dementia
if we have to courage to look across our borders,
if we have the courage to believe that we've always
had the answer
and we just need to find it again.
But above all if we have the courage to lose...

I believe that in order to make gains as human beings we
should have the courage to lose.
The courage to lose the notions we're so desperately
clinging to,
the courage to acknowledge that the road we're travelling
isn't taking us to our destination
and the courage to believe that a different world is possible.

How bad can it be to lose a system that excludes people?

How bad is such a loss when freedom and dignity
take its place?

Can we still speak of a loss in that case?

I believe that if we have the courage to lose,
those that matter stand to gain.

#HumanForever

Acknowledgements

We're filled with gratitude when we think about the very many people who made it possible for us to embark on this journey. It's in no small part thanks to you that we were able to realise our dream and that we felt supported every step of the way. Before we single out a few individuals, we'd like to thank all the wonderful people who played a part in this adventure from the bottom of our heart. Thank you for your stories, for your help in difficult times, for your openness, for your wise lessons, incisive analyses, the insights and contacts you shared with us, but above all we'd like to thank you for your faith in us, in this mission, and the confidence you instilled in us.

There are some people who played a special role in this journey, and we'd like to take this opportunity to give them all the credit they deserve. First of all, Jonathan's family and in particular Inge Geerdink (his girlfriend), who spent three years doing everything possible to make sure our adventure was a success. You sacrificed so much and gave even more. We can't thank you enough. We'd also like to express our admiration for Jonathan's children Juliette, Bastus and Cato, who had to go without their father for long spells of time yet always waited cheerfully and patiently for us to return. We love you.

And of course we can't leave out Teun's housemates. Therefore, I would like to thank them for the remarkable friendships and love over the years. Dear Ad †, Leny †, Muriëlle †, Tineke †, Elly †, Juul, Marjan, Piet †, Eugenie †, Clara †, Lambert †, Janna †, Nel †, Teunie †, Jeanne and Ida †, Wil, Janny, Jopie, Christel and Ko †, I'll carry you and all the fun, special and touching moments in my heart forever.

Someone else who's very dear to us and who has backed our mission from the outset is our good friend Bastiaan Brand. Not only did he play an essential role in the making of the documentary, but he's also always happy to help, in any way possible. You're a real pillar of strength to us. Because of your role behind the scenes not many people are aware of this, but know that we appreciate you all the more. For that reason we also want to thank your girlfriend Stephanie and daughter Bobbie for their patience with us.

We'd also like to thank our friends and families for their loving support. We hope to make up for the missed time together in the years to come.

Our thanks, too, to residential care homes Voorhoeve and Groenelaan and care organisations AxionContinu and Amstelring for their courage and trust in us by opening up their world and with it that of many of their residents. It's so cool that you gave Teun the chance to live on the secure unit and be a voice for those who are so rarely heard. It was a brave move, but it also shows a vulnerability and a willingness to improve the future of healthcare. Special thanks also to both the professional and informal caregivers.

To all the other people we spoke to for this book, wherever you are in the world: thank you for the inspiration. We're committed to sharing your stories and messages with as many people as possible worldwide, in a way that does justice to the range of different experiences of dementia, while stressing how valuable each individual one is. With the help of you and your stories we can challenge the dominant narrative of loss and show that if we change our perspective on people in general and people with dementia in particular, a more hopeful and more inclusive world is closer than we think.

We would also like to thank Elik Lettinga at De Arbeiderspers and Paulien Loerts at Singel Uitgeverijen for their faith in our second book. Our editor Esther Hendriks for overseeing the project and Jasper Velzeboer for dotting the i's and crossing the t's.

Finally, we'd like to thank all the individuals and institutions that supported and inspired us: we could never have done all this without your help. Thank you to the people and organisations from:

- THE NETHERLANDS – Henk Nies, AxionContinu, Martin den Hartog, Marie-Claire van Hek, Zorggroep Apeldoorn, Margje Mahler, Landgoed Grootenhout, Francien van de Ven, Noudje van Bussel, Doris van Vuuren, Huis van de Tijd, Anne-Mei The, Wonen bij September, Michiel van Putten, Huize Hunderen, Jose Driessen, Amstelring, Inge Borghuis, Jeroen Lambriks, Aunt Louise, Marcha Kwisthout, De Wever, Chantal Beks, Vivium Zorggroep, Jeanette Spiering, Anne-Margriet Pot, Rina Knippenberg, the Ministry of Health, Welfare and Sport, PGGM, Vilans, ActiZ, Alzheimer Nederland, V&VN, Zorgverzekeraars Nederland, Health and Youth Care Inspectorate, Dutch Health Care Authority, National Health Care Institute, Moniek

Beekx, Hans Toebes, Giel Toebes, Joep Toebes, Lieve Toebes and Moeder (grandma) Beekx, Wouter de Jong, Wiesje Houweling, Emaan de Jong, Jehuda de Jong, Aram de Jong, Chawwa de Jong, Thabije de Jong, Christiaan de Jong, Mechteld Prijs, Constantijn Prijs, Olivier Prijs, Johan and Els Geerdink.

- BELGIUM – All the residents at the nursing homes, Huis Perrekes, Carla Molenberghs, WZC Aymonshof, Tanja Everaert, Patricia Bauters, WZC De Weister, Jan Goddaer, Dirk Doucet, Kris Matuscsak, Paul van Tendeloo, Gudrun Callewaert and Jan van Wezer.
- MOLDOVA – All the residents at psychiatric hospital Orhei, the Ministry of Health, Labor and Social Protection, the cities of Chişinău and Grebleşti, the village of Calfa, Marcella Zbigli, Piotr †, Aliona Chricu, Petru Stratan, Ludmila Ceaglic, Andrei Pirgaru, Gheorghe Cornea.
- SOUTH KOREA – Ministry of Health and Welfare, First Vice Minister Yang Sung-Il, Member of Congress Jonghean Baek, the cities of Seoul and Busan, Team Superbrain, Solomon Han, Soyoung Moon, Jeehyang Jeong, Changhyung Hong, Hee Kyung Park, Seong Hye Choi, Hee Kyung Park, Seong Hye Choi.
- NORTH AMERICA – the state of Ohio, the city of Cleveland, Intergenerational School Cleveland, Case Western Reserve University Cleveland, Peter Whitehouse, Danny George, Pia Kontos, Teepa Snow, Al Power and Bry Weathly.
- SOUTH AFRICA – the cities of Cape Town, George and Mossel Bay, Aunt Gloria, Tommy Gozongo, Arlene Seconds, David Seconds, Rayne Stroebel, Adele van Wyk, Jaco Hofmann, Marguerite Schneider, Izak Niehaus, Celeste de Jager, Sebastiana Kalula and Henry Spencer.

- DENMARK – All the residents at the various nursing homes, Plejecenter Hundested, Mette Sofie Haulrich, Dagmarsminde, May Bjerre Eiby, Anneke Dapper.
- SWEDEN – the city of Stockholm, Karolinska Institute, World-Wide FINGERS Network, Miia Kivipelto, Sigrid Eklof and Petra Tegman.
- NORWAY – Stavanger Kommune, Stokka Sykehjem, Irene Todnem Hiis, Henriette Stavnem, Ruth-Karin Haslerud and Rita Weum.
- SLOVENIA – Ministry of Health, the city of Ljubljana, Zvezdan Pirtošek, Milica Gregorič Kramberger, Stefania Zlobec, Spomincica and David Krivec.
- UNITED KINGDOM – Gill Livingston, September Publishing, Hannah MacDonald, READ Media and Katie Read.
- GERMANY – Alexander Kurz, Lea Pfaffel.
- SWITZERLAND – the town of Balstahl, residential nursing home Lindenpark, Gina Kunst.
- CHINA – Andre Jager.
- INDIA – Sridhar Vaitheswaran, Zarin Gupta, Stichting Nightingale.
- NIGERIA – Kikelomo Laniyonu Edwards, Temitope Farombi, Josephine Anenih.
- KENYA – Wanjiku Joyce Kairu.
- GUINEA – Kadiatou Karouma, Aly Traore.
- BOLIVIA – Anita Badani.
- ITALY – Marcello Galetti.
- SPAIN – Laura Westers and Marcelo Diaz.
- BOSNIA AND HERZEGOVINA – Osman Kucuk.
- NORTH MACEDONIA – Gabriela Novotni.
- SLOVAKIA – Sabine Gergely, Maria Čunderlikova, Alexandra Palkovič.
- BULGARIA – Ivo Popivanov.

Ethical considerations

In *Human Forever* we use a rhizomatic-narrative approach to explore what a better life for people with dementia might look like. Rhizome thinking is based on the principle that people don't have just a single life story. In addition to the story that's highlighted at a specific moment in time there are many others. Or as the French philosopher Jean-François Lyotard put it: 'Being prepared to receive what thought is not prepared to think is what deserves the name of thinking.'

The idea for this book came out of the documentary *Human Forever*. The two are closely connected, as are the protagonists of both. All the people who feature in the publication gave us explicit permission to record and include their stories for the documentary, for which we're very grateful. We couldn't fit all the experiences into the film but seeing that it would be a shame to let their valuable contributions go to waste we decided to include them in a book, on the understanding that their consent for the visual image also applies to the less immediately recognisable written representation of their story.

Out of respect for the people with dementia, we have retained their own words and perceptions, even when they couldn't have any basis in fact. We respected everybody's privacy, and when someone (or their legal guardian) told us they didn't want to be in the book, we anonymised them and changed any identifying features. Because we attach great importance to the autonomy of people living with dementia, Teun asked his housemates for permission first. Only then did he turn to their legal guardians (who were often their children).

The conversations in countries with a language other than Dutch were conducted in English and German, or through an interpreter. We proceeded on the assumption that both the translations and the interpretations of feelings by the interpreter were accurate.

Our views, opinions and statements are informed by our own experiences and should never be regarded as *the* truth, but as *our* truth. On occasion we deliberately said things in a less nuanced way to better convey a point. Given that there's almost always an exception to the rule, we carefully weighed our words at every turn.

Not a word in this book is intended as a personal reproach, and we would like to distance ourselves in advance from any accusation by third parties that calls that into question.

We consulted research data from scholars from different scientific and cultural backgrounds from the following countries: the Netherlands, Belgium, Germany, England, Sweden, Norway, Finland, Denmark, France, Spain, Italy, Slovakia, Bulgaria, Romania, North Macedonia, Moldova, Slovenia, Serbia, Saudi-Arabia, Cyprus, Greece, Switzerland, Nigeria, Kenya, Ghana, Guinea, South Africa, Bolivia, Colombia, Argentina, Brazil, the United States, Canada, China, India and South Korea.

We received a great deal of help from Francien van de Ven, Anne-Mei The, Michiel van Putten, Anne Margriet Pot, Margje Mahler, Henk Nies, Carla Molenberghs, Jan Goddaer, Dirk Doucet, Kris Matuscsak, Paul van Tendeloo, Gudrun Callewaert, Jan van Wezer, Tanja Everaert, Patricia Bauters, Marcella Zbigli, Piotr +, Aliona Chricu, Petru Stratan, Ludmila Ceaglic, Andrei Pirgaru, Gheorghe Cornea, Solomon Han, Soyoung Moon, Jeehyang Jeong, Changhyung Hong, Hee Kyung Park, Seong Hye Choi, Peter Whitehouse, Danny George, Pia Kontos, Teepa Snow, Al Power, Bry Weathly, Rayne Stroebel, Adele van Wyk, Jaco Hofmann, Henry Spencer, Mette Sofie Haulrich, May Bjerre Eiby, Anneke Dapper, Miia Kivipelto, Sigrid Eklof, Petra Tegman, Gill Livingston, Irene Todnem Hiis, Henriette Stavnem, Ruth-Karin Haslerud, Rita Weum, Zvezdan Pirtošek, Milica Gregorič Kramberger, Stefania Zlobec, David Krivec, Alexander Kurz, Lea Pfaffel, Gina Kunst, Andre Jager, Sridhar Vaitheswaran, Zarin Gupta, Kikelomo Laniyonu Edwards, Temitope Farombi, Josephine Anenih, Wanjiku Joyce Kairu, Kadiatou Karouma, Aly Traore, Anita Badani, Marcello Galetti, Laura Westers, Marcelo Diaz, Sabine Gergely, Maria Čunderlikova, Alexandra Palkovič, Gabriela Novotni, Osman Kuck and Ivo Popivanov.

We assume that our contacts shared their oral and written information with us in good faith, not least because many of the researchers we interviewed are at the forefront of scientific research and have led studies that have been published in highly respected scientific publications.

None of the locations or people were paid to participate, and we didn't accept gifts, donations or bribes to visit places and include or exclude certain perspectives.

Finally, all the stories in this book are true, but occasionally we tweaked the time, place and order in which they took place to aid the narrative. We have done our utmost to present facts and source references as comprehensively as possible.

Sources

World Health Organisation (WHO), Dementia – key facts
https://www.who.int/news-room/fact-sheets/detail/dementia

The Lancet, 'Forecasting the prevalence of dementia'
https://www.thelancet.com/journals/lanpub/article/PI-IS24682667(21)00277-2/fulltext

The Netherlands, Fact sheet on dementia
https://www.alzheimer-nederland.nl/factsheet-cijfers-en-feiten-over-dementie

www.zorgcijfersdatabank.nl is the database on healthcare facts and figures from the National Health Care Institute of the Netherlands. The institute receives a great deal of data that allows it to properly carry out its various statutory tasks. This includes financial data and health insurance claim data from health insurers and care administration offices. Using its extensive knowledge of the healthcare system, the institute analyses these data flows to get a better understanding of cost developments in care.

The Netherlands, 'What matters most: Exploring the everyday lives of people with dementia' https://onlinelibrary.wiley.com/doi/10.1002/gps.5983

Belgium, dementia data
https://www.dementie.be/home/wat-is-dementie/prevalentie/

Scandinavia, 'Nordic Healthcare: Why Scandinavians are so healthy?'
https://www.dailyscandinavian.com/nordic-healthcare-why-scandinavians-
are-so-healthy/

Sweden, 'Swedish healthcare is largely tax-funded. And the overall quality is high'
https://sweden.se/life/society/healthcare-in-sweden

Worldwide FINGERS method https://fbhi.se/world-wide-fingers-network/

The Lancet, 'Dementia prevention, intervention, and care: 2020 report of the Lancet Commission'
https://www.thelancet.com/article/S0140-6736(20)30367-6/fulltext

The Lancet, 'Dementia Prevention in memory clinics: recommendations from the European task force for brain health services'
https://www.thelancet.com/journals/lanepe/article/PIIS26667762(22)00272-1/fulltext

South Africa, 'Storying Elderliness in Hangberg: a critical rhizolinguistic narrative journey'
https://dspace.stir.ac.uk/handle/1893/34641

South Africa, 'World Population Ageing'
https://www.un.org/en/development/desa/population/publications/pdf/ageing/WPA2017_Highlights.pdf

South Africa, 'Protecting South Africa's Elderly'
https://www.statssa.gov.za/?p=13445

South Africa, 'Townships in the South African Geograph-ic Landscape – Phyiscal and Social Legacies and Challenges'
https://www.treasury.gov.za/divisions/bo/ndp/ttri/ttri%20oct%202007/day%201%20-%2029%20oct%202007/1a%20keynote%20address%20li%20pernegger%20paper.pdf

'South Korea to become world's most aged country in 2044: data'
https://www.chinadaily.com.cn/a/202209/05/WS6315b3d-5a310fd2b29e7604c.html

TEAM SUPERBRAIN, 'Impact of multi-domain life-style intervention on cerebral cortical thickness and serum-brain-derived neurotrophic factor: the SUPERBRAIN exploratory sub-study'
https://www.ncbi.nlm.nih.gov/pmc/articles/PMC9606175/

TEAM SUPERBRAIN, 'Impact of a multi-domain lifestyle intervention on white matter integrity: The SUPERBRAIN exploratory sub-study'
https://www.frontiersin.org/articles/10.3389/fnagi.2023.1242295/full

TEAM SUPERBRAIN, https://www.rowan.kr/en_index. php

United States, Intergenerational School, https://www.ig-schools.org/

United States, Peter Whitehouse, ed. 'Concepts of Alzheimer Disease. Biological, Clinical, and Cultural Perspectives', https://www.press.jhu.edu/books/title/1351/concepts-alzheimer-disease

The Netherlands, Sociale Benadering Dementie (social approach to dementia)
https://socialebenadering.nl/

The Netherlands, Huis van de Tijd (House of Time) https://www.huisvandetijd.nu/

The Lancet, 'Overcoming the social death of dementia through language.'
https://www.thelancet.com/journals/lancet/article/PIIS014067361061286X/fulltext